Nursing
by
Heart

Transformational Self-Care
for Nurses

Nursing by Heart

Transformational Self-Care
for Nurses

Julie Skinner

AYNI BOOKS

Winchester, UK
Washington, USA

First published by Ayni Books, 2015
Ayni Books is an imprint of John Hunt Publishing Ltd., Laurel House, Station Approach,
Alresford, Hants, SO24 9JH, UK
office1@jhpbooks.net
www.johnhuntpublishing.com
www.ayni-books.com

For distributor details and how to order please visit the 'Ordering' section on our website.

Text copyright: Julie Skinner 2014

ISBN: 978 1 78279 711 1
Library of Congress Control Number: 2014945523

A CIP catalogue record for this book is available from the British Library.

Design: Stuart Davies

Printed and bound by CPI Group (UK) Ltd, Croydon, CR0 4YY

We operate a distinctive and ethical publishing philosophy in all
areas of our business, from our global network of authors to
production and worldwide distribution.

CONTENTS

Foreword

Many of us live in fear, trying to appease others, unable to connect to our heart's inner knowing. It is not often that we are presented with a guide that makes this process seem achievable.

I had worked with Julie for almost a decade in a harsh medical setting where both patients and staff often felt threatened, powerless, frustrated and frightened. Despite the oppressive environment, Julie stood out as a nurse whose skill, compassion and apparent patience appeared to define the best qualities of nursing that earned her the respect of her nursing and medical colleagues. However, as with many of us, Julie's demeanor during the early years often belied her insecurities and her self-doubt about her inherent strengths that were obvious to others.

Nursing by Heart is the culmination of the lessons, strategies and truths that have cultivated Julie's emotional and spiritual growth to become a truly confident, peaceful and fulfilled person who remains connected to her personal values and who inspires trust and hope in others. Infused with appropriate brief references to her own life journey, Julie's writing style is accessible to everyone. It educates as it awakens the reader's own inner truths. It stimulates the heart as it soothes the mind.

Coming to terms with our feelings in challenging life-situations is usually confronting. *Nursing by Heart* surprises as it addresses the strategies to these issues in a gentle and loving manner that is comforting yet enlightening. It makes the complex simple to understand.

In our service to others over our lifetime, we can become detached, burnt out and dissatisfied with life. In a cynical world full of self-help books, self-advancement seminars and clichéd leadership forums, *Nursing by Heart* stands apart as a guide that teaches its reader how to reach that heartfelt inner knowing that resides within each of us and inspires our lives. I would endorse its value to every nurse, to every doctor, to every helping professional, indeed to every person. The first person we need to nurse is ourselves.

Dr Tony Mastroianni
Senior Consultant Psychiatrist

Foreword

As nurses we are constantly required to adapt. We practice in a wide variety of environments but, wherever we are, competing priorities are a way of life. The vagaries of economic rationalism, striving to provide the best possible care for our patients, deciding what evidence-based best practice is, Key Performance Indicators ... to name a few. All compete for our attention at work and then there are family and friends, study and much more.

All this 'busy' overshadows the importance both personally and professionally of stopping, reflecting and listening to our own hearts.

Julie's book is a distillation of her years of experience within clinical nursing practice. It is gently written in a style that reflects the author's demeanor. *Nursing by Heart* contributes to the written work that reflects the awareness that nursing is a combination of art, science, heart and soul work.

Entwined within its reflective narrative are facets of Julie's professional journey through clinical practice and various nursing roles. It is always a pleasure for me to read thoughts on nursing written by a nurse for a nurse. I will no doubt dip back into *Nursing by Heart*. It is like a cool drink on a hot day.

It was just what I needed to read and I expect that will be true for many nurses who read it.

Marcia Sherring
Clinical Nurse Consultant
—commenced nursing June 1976 and still nursing May 2014

Foreword

This is a wonderfully timely book.

While nurses have more career opportunities than ever before, they also have never been under more pressure. Self-care is more important than it has ever been, in this fast-paced modern world we live in, and yet it is usually what is most likely to fall by the wayside.

As a psychologist I am all too aware of the dangers of burnout, and the impact it has both on the professional, and those they interact with. I see it in clients I work with, and those in my own profession. Nurses also have chosen to enter a helping profession, and they, like other helpers, tend to be most focused on caring for others, often not noticing their own needs until they are totally depleted.

Unfortunately the training they receive, though comprehensive in many areas, is largely bereft of recommendations and ideas on this vital topic, usually leaving it as simply making sure you take some time for yourself. While this is good advice, by itself it is not particularly useful, and people are often left wishing their days and weeks away, longing for the weekend or the end of their shift, feeling burnt out, depressed and ineffectual.

Far better is the approach recommended in Julie's book: taking an active part in what we offer in service to others, without depleting ourselves. Imagine if we could actively love our jobs, taking the challenges of the workplace in our stride. Imagine if we could feel confident of the service we offer without feeling responsible for our patients' choices and outcomes, and without giving in to self-doubt or leaving ourselves feeling wrung out and exhausted! What a relief that would be and what space that would grant to those of us who help others, allowing us to simply give without expectation, of either the client's outcome or our own ability to be 'useful.'

I wholeheartedly recommend this book to nurses, and indeed anyone who chose a profession that is about helping others, as a way to rediscover your passion in your work, to remember why you chose this field, what it means to be a professional helper and to again feel the joy to be found in working with people.

Claudia Vayda
Psychologist

Acknowledgments

This book would not have been created if not for the encouragement and ongoing love and support of my mentors Michael and Segolene King of the Cosmosis Mentoring Centre. They champion my spirit.

I thank the early readers of my manuscript, Claudia and Kim, who offered great suggestions. My editor Laura Daniel skillfully and respectfully fostered structure and clarity from the initial manuscript.

I have much gratitude to Linda Koen for her compassion and wisdom, seeing me through some tough times.

I appreciate the unique gifts of Nerida, modeling Humility in action.

To the many friends that inspire my heart with their courage and generosity: Debbie, Belinda, Patti, Karen, Marguerite, Liljana, Debbie, Simon, Arlene and Rupert.

A special acknowledgment to Asifa who lovingly kept me accountable during the completion of the final draft.

Thank you to my children, Andrei and Lana, who both inspire me to be a better person. I am kinder and more selfless for their presence in my life.

I have been graced with some special people in my life and Paul Spurr is one such; one who believed in me and quietly encouraged me to develop my reflective gifts many years ago. The world of Reflective Clinical Supervision benefits from his contribution.

There are many talented facilitators I have had the pleasure to work with and I extend a special thank-you to Michelle Eason who was instrumental in my move to the facilitation world. I remember fondly Michelle, Karen, Ketty and Sheree for their ongoing dedication to bringing in the new.

I dedicate this book to my mother Pat who passed away

recently. She embodied a quiet, determined presence and taught me that things are often not as they seem.

Thank you to all the wonderful nurses I have known and indeed all in the caring profession who offer kind, compassionate care, making a difference to patients' lives.

Chapter 1

What Would It Be Like If...?

What lies behind us and what lies before us are tiny matters compared to what lies within us.
~ Ralph Waldo Emerson

A revolution in nursing is transforming how nurses practice their profession.

Nurses are some of the hardest-working people I know. We are practical, decisive, and organized with an inherent desire to care for others. The art and science of nursing need to be one, where compassionate care is as prized as the knowledge and skill to deliver expert care. But nurses are exhausted, burnt out and frustrated. Nurses need to know how to care for themselves on a deeper level than what is currently on offer—the usual self-care advice. Self-care is multifaceted, but care of the spirit can't be ignored for true self-care to exist.

The old transactional model wherein nurses followed directions from others, with little of their own input, is being laid to rest—the end of the old paradigm. The old hierarchical structure no longer serves the needs of the health system or recognizes the expertise of nurses as the greatest resource in any hospital. This presents a challenge for some aspects of the nursing profession, as we are encouraged and expected to have a voice, share ideas, and create new models of care; but perhaps we are still constrained by the old and resistant to this new level of responsibility.

An intense focus on nursing in recent times has encouraged transformation of the way we practice nursing. I have had the pleasure and privilege of being part of that change, as both facilitator of a leadership program and trainer of a reflective clinical supervision program, working alongside other wonderfully skilled facilitators who have a vision for nursing wherein all health professionals within teams are empowered to deliver the best possible care. For empowered teams to work, each member must be recognized as having a contribution to make to its health and functioning.

I offer here a perspective that has not been explicitly addressed in this transformational movement but is very much present in all we do as humans. I present practical tools to incorporate into our practice, beginning with cultivation of a relationship with self—acknowledging ourselves as something much more than just physical beings. This allows us to explore who we really are—which is much more than what we perceive—and to build from the strongest foundation possible.

Empowering the self changes how we engage with others. Raising awareness of how we are in the world and of the impact we create fosters new opportunities for behaviors that are self-loving and attract others to want to work with us.

With the health dollar shrinking, our traditional resources are under pressure, and workloads are a constant concern for nurses, but our relationships with others are underdeveloped, and these are our richest resource. I have often heard nurses exclaim that their difficulties in the workplace come from other nurses, not from caring for patients. This situation is not peculiar to nursing, as our relationships with others constantly challenge us to find ways to connect with others to understand each other.

Why is this book so different from others? It acknowledges that each of us embodies the potential to transform self, our practice and our relationships with others by addressing what is at the heart of our profession, seeing ourselves in a fuller sense.

We are energetic beings, and we can manage our energy field through understanding this and learning to be more conscious of how we fundamentally engage with others. We live in a sea of energy—to which we and others contribute—the energy that

9

bathes us on this planet.

Imagine what it would be like to be able to manage our own energy field rather than to be at the mercy of what others project onto us. I invite you to feel the implications for our nursing practice as we envision a future wherein each of us takes responsibility for what we emote or share energetically with others.

I have been nursing for more than thirty years and feel excited to be part of this change. We will all benefit. Patients will experience the best possible care, as we relate to them by honoring their wholeness, not just their physical being. They will be respected as the experts of their care, and they will be cared for by cohesive teams of people who value creativity and collaboration, bringing forth collective knowledge and wisdom. Each of us will bring a unique voice to the delivery of care, and each will be acknowledged for her or his unique contribution. The organizations and institutions that employ us will benefit from a profession driving change that impacts one and all.

This new paradigm differs greatly from what I experienced as a young second-year nursing student in 1984. I was on a three-month placement in the Intensive Care Unit in a large teaching hospital in Adelaide, South Australia. I was rostered on ten consecutive night shifts after a week of day shifts. When I questioned this, I was told this was the usual rostering practice and 'just the way it was.' This acceptance of a practice that was potentially dangerous to both the nurses and the patients in their care puzzled me. I wondered then, and often again over the years, what drove this acceptance. At the time, I braced myself for the long nights ahead and did my best to stay awake on the forty-minute drive home, windows down, eating fruit or sugary foods, willing myself to concentrate on the winding roads climbing the Adelaide Hills. I was so exhausted by the eighth night that I rang the supervisor in tears to say I couldn't come in, sharing honestly the reasons. I was told I must report for duty as rostered unless I was sick and had a doctor's certificate.

This taught me that as a nurse I wasn't valued and that the needs of others were always to come first. There was no understanding that my welfare was related to the care I could provide for patients. I believe this rostering system was a part of nursing training, designed to produce nurses who followed directions. Parallels with the military were evident. I remember thinking what a strange system I worked in, given that nurses were the backbone of hospitals. We were trained to have diverse skills and to expertly care for very ill patients, yet we were treated like naughty school children. This seemed to create a culture of blame, as, when people believe they are without influence, they can direct the energy of frustration and resentment towards each other. I am sure that we can all recall an experience of this, and perhaps, driven by frustration, we have originated such behavior.

I am curious to know how this hospital-based training continues to impact us today.

How much impact does this have on how we support new nurses entering the profession?

How can we contribute to empowering nurses to value themselves and others, and what influence can we have on our profession by embedding new ways of nursing practice?

A year after completing my training, I decided I wasn't cut out for general nursing. I enjoyed the diversity of the experience and making a difference in the lives of patients, but I felt suffocated by the oppressive culture. I was attracted to Mental Health Nursing, believing it offered a different experience wherein diversity was accepted and nurses were encouraged to have a viewpoint, as there was less certainty in this specialty area. My belief turned out to be somewhat true and somewhat false. There was, indeed, a greater acceptance of diversity, and nurses were more encouraged to express their views, but those views could be judgmental, reflecting the unresolved aspects of each of us—

saying more about the person expressing the view than about the patient.

I became more interested in how I could help the patient without imposing my own bias and unresolved issues. I seemed to find my niche, and I stayed in Mental Health for more than twenty years, training in one of the original psychiatric institutions in Sydney, Australia then working for six years in an acute admission unit in the inner city and, later, caring for mentally ill patients in jail.

Within healthcare settings, there is growing interest in working with the principles of collaboration and engagement, fostering well-functioning teams in which each member accesses her own knowledge and brings it together with that of others, in respect and consideration, to create team empowerment. The challenge I see for nurses is in fostering a strong belief in self— the confidence to find, and express from, a space of liberation, breaking free of the limitations of the old paradigm, building internal resources and creating a new box of tools to draw upon in the practice of nursing.

Teaching nurses the importance of caring holistically for the self is foundational; and giving care to patients from a space of fullness rather than depletion is essential for the profession. Increasingly scarce resources in healthcare is a real issue, but we have a wealth of resources in human potential. Can you imagine what nursing will be like when each of us taps into our own potential, finding the creativity and innovation within?

Pondering the changes I have seen and experienced during my thirty years of nursing, I am truly amazed. I didn't imagine I would be working in management or education, as I was reserved by nature and didn't believe I had much to offer. I decided to stop allowing this to be an impediment to sharing my gifts and decided to stop hiding away, waiting to be perfect and instead have a go. This has helped me assist others to discover their unique gifts, as not feeling ready is a common experience.

This difficulty is something I have acknowledged and continue to heal in myself, and I can nurture and offer a genuineness, an authenticity, in relating to others.

Genuineness or authenticity is much more than this, but this is a great starting point, taking our true selves wherever we go, not creating different masks according to the people we are with, trying to fit into a box others have created for us. Believing that we need many different masks to effectively relate to different people is an illusion cultivated by not believing we are enough; so we cover, distort and build layers over our core essences. We can remove these veils we have created, freeing ourselves from illusion, finding the truth of who we really are.

What if there were nothing wrong with any of us, nothing that needed fixing, rather it is simply a choice to remove the veils of illusion that cover our inner radiance?

Fixing others or feeling responsible for others becomes redundant, as there is nothing wrong with any of us, nothing that needs fixing in the way we may believe.

How can we assist others to see, discovering their radiant essence?

By expressing from the heart, courageously daring to be vulnerable, sharing what we believe in, what we value, and not judging others for their choices.

As nurses, we tend to be very good problem solvers and are trained to make decisions quickly and constantly in the delivery of patient care. This makes giving advice very much second nature to us. The busyness of most wards has allowed limited time for or encouragement of reflection on our professional practice. This reluctance to reflect on our practice is what impedes us, as we are very skilled at task completion but not so skilled at valuing our knowledge and informing other health professionals what we do. However, we can raise awareness of who we are as nurses only from reflection on our practice and thus discover new and innovative ways of caring for self and others.

An example of how to begin to do this is to reflect with intent and commitment at the end of a shift, acknowledging what went well and what could be improved. This honest retrospection strengthens our ability to reflect in the moment next time, giving us something new to draw on. This process, practiced consistently, develops skills for being more fully present in each moment.

One way we can learn to empower self and others is to discern when giving advice is desirable and when there is an opportunity for others to find their own way. Asking questions that assist self-exploration offers others a development tool. When I have missed an opportunity and have given advice to another rather than asking some enabling questions, I know I have disempowered that person, holding her in a limiting belief that she could not find a way forward. I may have done this because I was busy and giving the answer is quicker, or I may enjoy feeling important as the bearer of knowledge.

What does this bring up for you?

What if each of us knows what is best for self and that we can best assist others not by giving advice but by asking questions, enabling them to access the knowing within?

All skills can be learnt and enhanced when we see value in their application. Several years ago, new to my role as a Nursing Unit Manager, I believed that solving the team's problems was my responsibility. In retrospect, I see that in dispensing quick answers I felt validated as a new manager, reasoning that if I knew the answers, I was deserving of the role. Nonetheless, I felt conflicted in this role I had created—being the holder of knowledge—as I was so busy assisting the nurses I managed I often needed to stay late to understand and complete the paperwork from my new role. 'Needing to be needed' is a powerful driver for many of us, and this pattern disempowers others because we create dependency. If others no longer need us to solve their problems, how can we have our need satisfied? I felt a weight lift when I came to understand this and began instead to practice the art of questioning to enable others to make their own decisions by encouraging and allowing, recognizing their potential and most importantly healing this pattern within myself.

I learnt how to better assist the team to acknowledge their strengths and to develop weaker areas by asking enabling questions when I was presented with the day-to-day issues of the ward. I knew that many of the team knew how to address the various issues, but some lacked the confidence to enact their ideas, or some were just being lazy thinkers. Some felt surprised that they actually did know how to move forward; however, some were occasionally frustrated, as they had been accustomed to coming to me for answers and were then being asked for their own ideas.

It was also frustrating for me, as working in a more enabling way initially took longer as I needed to stop and consider how to do this. We can all get caught up in the busyness of the day and forget to be future focused. The rewards were evident down the track, as some of the team would come to me to discuss their ideas that would then be taken back to the team for a trial. The team were more engaged in decisions and knew they would be listened to. A breakthrough came one day when a young nurse came to see me and said: 'I know you are going to ask me what I would like to do about this, so I have an idea.' I felt heartened as this seemed the beginning for this nurse to try a new way, and I watched her flourish over the years, learning the value of enabling questions and using them in her own practice.

Imagine what it would be like if enabling others were embraced in teams across our hospitals?

The health dollar is stretched to breaking point, and adequate funding, although important, is only a part of the solution. We need to understand that we are each a part of the solution if we embrace all of our gifts and take responsibility for what is within our level of influence by accessing and putting to practical use much more of who we really are.

To all who can hear by listening with their hearts and feeling the ancient wisdom encouraging us to step forward, to take action, know that we are not buffeted by the winds of fate but are instead able to create whatever life we choose. We can learn to feel on all levels of our being, creating deeper levels of maturity and authenticity that inspire others as we respond rather than react to life.

How would you like to learn a way to fully engage with how you feel and to transform not only your nursing practice but your life?

Can you sense the strength and possibility in that for yourself and all in your sphere of influence?

Chapter 2

Self-Care at Its Heart

It is when you give of yourself that you truly give.
~ Kahlil Gibran

When we care for self at a deep level where spirit resides, we can give a most generous gift to others—the gift of self, in true service, from a clear and loving space, giving from the overflow.

As nurses, we have the collective potential to lead a transformation in the healthcare setting, as we are represented in large numbers, with a diverse range of skills, and are found in almost all places across the planet. When each of us focuses on working together to transform our area of influence, we can create a sea of change, where personal healing occurs at our own cores and ripples out to all within our environments.

Pivotal to this shift is to first explore our relationship with self, as this is foundational to all the relationships we have with others. Until we are honest with ourselves and raise our awareness of what drives our behaviors, we contribute to the fear that surrounds us, thus remaining part of the problem that limits and contracts our experiences and then our environments.

We are energetic beings, and everything is energy interfacing with energy. If this were recognized and accepted and taught, we could relate very differently. We could create well-functioning teams where each person took responsibility for their own behavior and sought to contribute their best.

A mushrooming of ideas in the last few years encourages us to become more aware of our thoughts so we can think more effectively, telling us we are what we think. Although much of this offers worthwhile ways to improve our relationship with self and others, it misses a vital understanding: We are much more than thinking bodies—we relate on many levels in a constant dance of energy. In order to have successful relationships with others, we need to first understand how to have integrity of our own energy field. By first relating better to ourselves and knowing who we are, we can build fuller relationships with others.

Nurses are used to operating on hunches; having a sense something isn't right. This is intuition at play where we just know

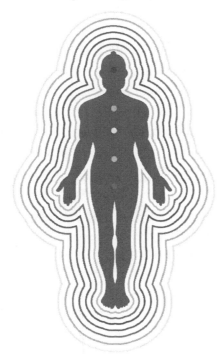

something, whether it be a patient needing assistance to get out of bed or a patient deteriorating. This is our higher senses at play as we are much more than thinking, physical bodies. We are spirit expressing through multiple energetic bodies that we don't sense in the same way as we do the physical body. The four-body system comprises the physical body, the emotional body, the mental body and the soul body. Then there are different levels within each of these bodies. Although we can't perceive these other bodies with our five senses, they can be accessed with our higher awareness. Knowing we are more than our physical bodies, we may have a sense of these other bodies. Or maybe we just have a sense of a larger area around our physical form. To have a sense of this we can feel into how we relate to others we don't know intimately. We generally maintain, and feel comfortable with, about a meter of space around our physical form. Could this preference we mostly have provide a way of appreciating how we experience energy? There are cultural aspects to this preference but, as an illustration, it may assist our understanding that we all emit an energetic charge and have an energetic signature that is as unique as our fingerprints. We can be attracted or repelled by the energy of others, depending on the quality of our own unique energy signature.

When we engage with others we create energetic cords or connections that form with others or things, and they keep us attached until we cut or clear them. These energy strands form every time we develop an attachment to something or someone and are the basis of feeling disempowered. The amount of 'stuff' we drag around accumulates over the years and can be substantial. Through our cord connections, we can be manipulated by others and we can manipulate others. Attachments will be further discussed in Chapter 7. Consider the last time you felt suddenly tired or depleted in someone's company or agreed to do something you didn't want to do. These experiences are common when we are corded with others. We can learn to clear these cords and maintain a clearer system to operate in. This is the basis of energetic hygiene and, practiced consistently over time, creates a lightness and vitality in our system that is deeply nourishing.

Can you imagine how it would be not to have washed for a long time and how good it would then feel to wash off all that debris?

* * *

Our four-body system accumulates energy from the fear in our surroundings, fear energy from others, and fear energy generated from within ourselves. Feel into how you are carrying all that old energy around. Just as energy can feel heavy and contracted, it can feel light and expansive at the other end of the scale. No wonder lethargy and tiredness are so commonly experi-enced. As nurses we are very accustomed to feeling this way after a shift. We can learn how to clear this energy we take on from others and not only assist ourselves but have more energy to care for others.

We can bring more love and light into our Being only by being present in our physical bodies, as it is through the physical body that we express as Spirit. There are many ways we can be not really present in our body. One way is a tendency to be dreamy and floaty, struggling to connect or relate to others or being distracted and misplacing personal belongings.

I invite you to engage in a process now to feel more grounded.

Take a few minutes to ground your energy now, feeling your connection to the earth beneath our feet, seeing and feeling roots of light, anchoring and stabilizing your system. Feel how different it is to ground ourselves and how it is then possible to bring more and more of self here into the present moment.

Aligning ourselves to the direction we are heading provides our first layer of energetic protection and our alignment can be visualized as a golden cylinder of light about a meter in circum-ference that infuses and surrounds the four-body system. Imagine this beautiful cylinder as a continuous column reaching out far above your head to deep within the earth. Now feel and see all your bodies lock into place over the heart, centering to allow us to express from the heart, connecting with the ground beneath our feet, deep into the earth.

It is common for us to think about how we are feeling rather than feeling how we are feeling. This moves energy out of the emotional body into the mental body, where it doesn't belong. We often also push unwanted feelings into the physical body, where they don't belong. Thus energy is displaced when we judge what we feel and don't want to acknowledge those feelings. This displacement of energy feels uncomfortable, and a lot of effort or energy is required to hold it all in place.

Do you have a sense of how this is for you?

We can get used to experiencing life this way and believe it is normal.

Imagine how it could be to regularly clear all that residue out by learning a process to let energy be where it is meant to be.

Just as we wash our physical bodies daily, so too it is important to clean our energetic bodies. We live in a dense realm where all kinds of fear dominate our surroundings, so we collect from other people and our environments these energetic projections. Have you ever felt completely drained after a shift and wondered whether it had to be that way?

Exhaustion is an experience nurses often feel at the end of a shift and if it continues over time, we can shut down our awareness of what we feel, running on empty. Nurses are empathic so easily pick up on others' feelings and want to help by unconsciously taking on the energy of others. This makes us prone to 'burnout' if we don't learn to clear our energy field. Burnout is a term that nurses understand well, either through experiencing it or being around other nurses who are living it. It is difficult for everyone to be around someone who is in a burnout state, as the person seems to have lost the ability to care and connect with self and therefore others. Learning to Ground your energy, Align to Spirit, and Centre in your heart and breath is the foundational way to connect us more deeply with others by first deepening the connection to self.

I invite you to feel for a moment how different our places of care could be if we all practiced this simple self-care strategy.

Rather than denying what we feel or judging our feelings as unacceptable, silly or invalid, we can really acknowledge what we are feeling. This does not mean to act upon our feelings by projecting them at others but, rather, to sit for a moment with the feeling, validating what is being felt, knowing that it may not be the truth of who we are, but it is valid. Rather than pushing our

feelings away, jamming up the physical body with unacknowl-
edged feelings or thoughts about our feelings, we can just
experience what we are feeling. It is such a relief to feel as we feel
without judgment, without filtering what we deem is okay to feel
and what should remain suppressed. Trying to control and filter
what we feel dams up energy and creates tension in our being.
Freeing up the energy, allowing it to flow, is its natural state, and
this can be achieved by all of us with consistent practice.

The next area to explore is how we identify what is our own
energy. If the energy has originated with you, then feeling it
without judgment is appropriate, but, if it is not, then we can
learn to let it go, to return to its rightful place.

Old coping behaviors that are not conducive to our ability to
deliver quality patient care or effective teamwork can be transformed, and this transformation is available to everyone, if we
choose to change our habits. Take a minute to consider whether
you would prefer a different experience, where you could feel
energized. Now imagine that you could release the judgment of
what you feel—either towards yourself or towards another.
Judgment keeps us stuck, sucking the life out of us. Judgment is
controlling and limiting, contracting our energy field and
rendering our energetic protection void—something we are very
used to doing. We are encouraged from a young age to judge, and
we call it critical thinking. How different might our experience be
if we practiced this simple self-care routine in our roles as
nurses? It can be challenging at first to practice this as we care for
others but, like anything, with consistent application, it becomes
part of our normal daily practice.

There is a common belief that emotions are feelings but this is
not the case. Emotions are more states of being that reside in the
emotional body. The emotional body is a body of energy that is a
part of our four-body system, whereas feelings are what we feel
and are designed to move through the four-body system to heal
and offer insight into our true selves. Feelings allow us to access

the heart's knowing, and as they are experienced on all levels of our being there is a richness in this experience. It is such a relief to feel as we feel without judgment. Letting go of trying to control and filter what we feel, we stop damming up energy, allowing more of it to flow through our system and, like a river, we are designed to flow with the energy allowing it to do what it was designed to do.

Nurses are care providers, caring for others, but we often have difficulty caring for ourselves. Even with an understanding of self-care, we may not always practice it. How would it be to end this disconnect and care for ourselves from the core level of our being? When we first take responsibility for our energetic field we have taken the first and most important step towards caring for ourselves as we no longer unconsciously take on energy that belongs to another. We can do this by clearing cords or energetic connections that we have with others.

Then we can take the next step — honoring what we feel, knowing that our feelings are the eyes to the heart — and begin to discover who we really are, not constrained by the voice of the inner critic that keeps us from being in all our radiance.

I used to be a 'fixer', feeling responsible for everything and everyone else, and I have observed many nurses following this same pattern. All professions hold unconscious programs, and nursing has a well-entrenched history of solving problems. It is useful to ask ourselves:

What need does this pattern fulfill within me?

The answer might help us understand what attracts us to certain professions and not others. In my case, this fixer pattern allowed me to validate myself, as I felt I valued helping others so it kept my focus on others. I was so busy fixing outside myself that I didn't have much time or energy left to focus on how I could develop myself.

When we seek validation outside of self, we do not trust our own navigator within—the voice of Spirit that guides our journey home. When we are focused on fixing others around us, we can use this as a distraction from that inner guidance. If each of us focused on being the best we could be and allowed others to make their choices, we would have a very different experience on this planet.

Can you imagine how that might be?

What a relief to let go of this and allow others to be as they choose and instead take responsibility for self, each of us being the best we can be.

Everything is energy, as energy is a wave-particle—unseen or as solid as a piece of wood—either loosely bound or tightly woven. When we engage with others, we share energy in many ways, especially as thoughts and feelings.

Consider how these scenarios are for you.

Feel into how you may experience a person who is dominant in her expression and imposes her views onto you. This can be experienced through the physical energetic body, maybe as a jolt to the solar plexus or an instant headache.

Hospitals tend to hold a dense energy, where the atmosphere feels heavy, as patients and their loved ones tend to be in a fear state, uncertain of outcomes and sensing the fragility of the physical form. When we are preoccupied, believing we are only thinking physical bodies, the fear of loss can be extreme. We are so much more than our thinking physical bodies, and when we choose to take responsibility for all our Being—physical, emotional, mental and soul—clearing and protecting our energetic field can be very freeing. We can choose what we allow into our field, maintaining our integrity, and thus assist others from a space of fullness rather than depletion.

Each of us is responsible for our own Being. We do not assist others by taking on their sadness, anger, anxiety or fear. Sympathy originates from the solar plexus—our center of human identification—and we are imagining how that situation would be for us if we were experiencing it, whereas empathy is a heartfelt union where we enter in vulnerability into another's world without attachment to the experience, just to be totally present for that person. As nurses, we are caring people, and we often unconsciously take on others' energy in a desire to assist. But it does not assist others to take on their energy; it disempowers them.

There is another way, if we learn to take responsibility for our own energetic field by practicing being grounded, present and feeling what is ours to feel without judgment. Before I learnt how to care for and protect my energy field, I was used to feeling tired most of the time during a shift and, after the shift ended, I just wanted to sleep. When, several years ago, I first started clearing my energetic field regularly, I felt a weight lifted from me, a sense of ease in my being and a great sense of relief. Now that I have practiced having much stronger boundaries, I can choose what I allow into my energy field and, when I forget, I can remember and re-strengthen my energetic boundaries. Then what I allow into my field becomes simply a choice. While learning, we need to be persistent and to practice, just as we do when we learn anything new. From this space of greater clarity, we can feel vital, more focused and settled in ourselves, able to be more of who we really are in each and every moment.

Nurses are carers, seeking to make a difference in the lives of others. We are part of that journey with patients as they travel the healthcare path. Sometimes the journey is fraught with discordant energies—the energy of fear. Fear is contagious. Ponder for a moment how, when someone around you is feeling fearful and anxious, that can very quickly become your reality. Until we learn energetic boundaries, we can be like sponges, absorbing the energies of those around us. As nurses, we sit more than most people in these dense, heavy energies, as hospitals hold the fear of patients and their families. Just as fear is contagious, so is the higher vibration—Calm Assurance, Hope and Compassion. These are sacred qualities and will be discussed in Chapter 4. We can assist others by holding a higher vibration of energy from a place of non-attachment and non-judgment, creating alternative possibilities for them. We can learn how and what energy to resonate with. It simply becomes a choice. Positive emotional states are also contagious and have the ability to raise the vibration of whole teams. Consider how a candle lights a room, no matter how dark.

You may be wondering: If this is true why are we not all doing it?

Why haven't we been taught this as children?

Because we have forgotten these ancient wisdoms, we have forgotten we have a choice. We have been taught instead to overvalue the lower mind, to rationalize and have an opinion on everything—which really teaches us how to judge. We have been taught not to feel thus can be uncomfortable with our feelings and the feelings of others. We have taken on beliefs that limit our expression.

I have noticed that feeling resentful is common among nurses, and I have certainly felt this, juggling so many demands without enough staff and feeling exhausted. Now when I feel resentment for all I have to do, I stop and take a moment to breathe and acknowledge what I am feeling rather than pushing on regardless. I feel grateful that I have noticed what I am feeling and prioritize what I need to do, focusing on being fully in the moment with each task. This helps me to come back into my center rather than scattering my energies. Then I can be fully present for another, where the other feels heard, their experience validated sending a message of: I value you and I'm listening to what you say.

Ponder the last time you did this for another and, even more importantly, for yourself.

To give each task our full attention drops the experience of feeling anxious as a default setting.

Feeling grateful for all we experience is the key to creating change in our lives and until we feel grateful for our experience we are pushing away that which we seek to attract. Being grateful for our experience means we are learning and growing from all we do rather than suffering our way through life.

Being grateful for our experiences is a component of emotional intelligence as when we are truly grateful we feel different, not like a victim to life. Quite a bit has been written about emotional intelligence, which simply means: the ability to respond rather than react, to be accountable for how we are with others as this contributes to the effect we create. Responding means taking responsibility for what is ours and not projecting it at another as a reaction. We don't react to others if we clear unconscious patterns, as reactions are those hurt parts of us coming to the fore and expressing because they have been activated.

Caring for self is not just our natural state of being but is a gift to others. When we give from a clear and loving space and hold another in this state of Compassion, we can truly assist another. Giving from a space of fullness and taking responsibility for our energetic field, monitoring the effect we evoke in others, is a very different experience to feeling like we are at the mercy of our circumstances, and everyone can learn this.

The process to clear and protect your energetic field is woven through this book. If you would like a daily version to practice please email me at julie@coretrue.com.au

Chapter 3

Bringing the Heart into Nursing

Nothing is softer or more flexible than water,
yet nothing can resist it.
~ Lao Tzu

A new paradigm in healthcare has emerged in the last few years and, although in its fledgling beginnings in most areas, it is gathering traction and a growing interest. We are all called to consider new ways to engage with others, valuing and respecting the contribution of each, creating inclusiveness. Collaboration builds engagement where each is a part of the greater whole and feels heard, creating clear communication and understanding. Given that most of our challenges in healthcare seem to have their basis in communication, if we can improve how we communicate with each other, the patient experience can only be enhanced.

When patients are surveyed to capture their satisfaction with service delivery, they usually voice the desire for a stronger human connection—a connection where they feel valued and heard as people, not merely as illnesses or injuries. Historically, nurses have been very good at treating the whole person in this way, but since elevating nursing to the status of 'profession', as indeed it is, there has been criticism that although we have grown professionally and our technical skills are much greater, the quality of our engagement with patients has declined.

The new paradigm is concerned with everyone's experience as, when we are 'person centered' rather than just 'patient centered', all are valued in the healthcare setting, and the experience for the collective is enhanced. Each shares a responsibility for the environment and owns her impact on the whole. Maybe we have experienced this and wondered how it could be if we are all prepared to explore courageously other ways of being in our health settings.

Engagement of all the team in a healthcare setting requires an exploration of roles and a genuine desire to share the decision-making. This can be very challenging for a manager, as it can be intoxicating to be the holder of knowledge and to have others seeking that knowledge. This can fulfill a pattern that many of us have running: a 'need to be needed'. As I shared briefly in the introduction, when we seek from others validation that we are worthy, we are attempting to fill a state of poor self-worth. Not feeling worthy is common for many people even when evidence to the contrary exists.

Until this is healed this pattern demands continuous fuel.

As a Nursing Unit Manager, I experienced this challenge, as I shared briefly in Chapter 1. It was assumed I had knowledge that others needed, and I was constantly asked to share that knowledge or to solve the team's problems. As I dispensed the knowledge and gave advice about all manner of problems, I felt my self-worth validated as I knew the answers. I was unsure if I could manage a team as I had no training for the role. However, I became increasingly frustrated, because I knew the staff had the ability to make many of these decisions themselves. I was also constantly interrupted as staff sought my advice, and as I struggled to complete the many demands of the role I often stayed late. I came to realize that not only was I depleting, I was disempowering the team; I suspected they had ideas they weren't sharing, or didn't trust their choices, or couldn't be bothered to think about a solution. However, part of me felt important and needed by my team and this, combined with the anxiety I felt as a new manager, was a potent mix. It was only when I built my worthiness, allowing confidence in the role to build, that I could do something different.

After several months, I decided to try something else as I had commenced a leadership program and learning new ways to engage with a team. I went about investigating how to manage a team in more enabling ways. I began asking individual team members what they thought about the problem they had brought to me and how they would like to solve it. There were mixed reactions as I was changing the goalposts, not routinely providing the answers. Some of the staff were annoyed, some delighted at being asked for their ideas, and some avoided bringing anything to me.

A better way may have been to engage the team in how they could share their ideas as I imposed this new way upon them. It may have been an improvement, but it did meet with considerable resistance. I could have had more of them buy into the strategy if the team had been asked how they would like to share their ideas. It is crucial that every person on a team have the opportunity to contribute, and this is really as simple as asking each person what they would like to share. This can create a sufficient shift for some teams, having a discernible effect on their functioning quite quickly. When people can say what they really think and feel, where transparency is valued and there is no fear of negative consequences, people can feel safe in contributing and exposing vulnerability.

* * *

Vulnerability is something most of us in healthcare shy away from, perhaps wanting to promote confidence that we know what we are doing as professionals and have the skills to assist patients back to optimum health. This reaction is valid as patients look to us for competence in our practice and reassurance. Vulnerability can be misunderstood though. We may use all our professional skills but not truly engage with a patient, and patients tell us this in patient surveys.

So what is Vulnerability? I see it as a strength; being in a state of honesty with self—expressing in authenticity, without pretense, not hiding what we are feeling but being as we are, in Acceptance and Respect for what we are feeling. From this space, we give others permission to do the same—connecting with another, allowing the other to experience connection with another feeling person, expanding and surrendering in a space of Vulnerability. To know there are many perspectives and we do not know the best way for others. When we pretend we know, steadfastly holding onto our mask of certainty, our energy expression can denote something quite different; we are really telling self and others that our feelings are not important and we don't feel okay in expressing how we feel. This can confuse others who may sense the incongruence, and we are promoting confusion to self and others. This is not about dumping our feelings onto others but is instead knowing we don't need to have all the answers as there are in Truth many perspectives and simply being honest with self and others allows another to access the right way for them.

Among facilitators, there is a divide where some believe that it is not okay to share how we are in a group, as maybe we are supposed to be the experts on subject content; but I believe the greatest gift we can give others is to take responsibility for what we are feeling so that we can step aside and not project our unresolved stuff onto another. There is Honesty in this as we are feeling how we are feeling without pretense. When we do this, we remove the masks we present to others. These masks protect us in a world that says it is not okay to feel. We wear these masks like a veneer, afraid to express our authentic self. When we value the Truth by being authentic, we build Trust and rapport with others more easily. Others can often perceive a disconnect between what we say and how we are actually expressing energetically.

How is this for you when another says 'I'm fine' but you feel their annoyance or distress? There is a way to build a bridge between these two states by modeling a new way.

I once listened to a speaker, an experienced presenter, begin his talk by sharing how anxious he felt. He turned his palms to the audience, showing us that his hands were dripping with sweat. He then went on to share both his love of public speaking and the topic he had prepared. In sharing this with his audience, he established rapport through sharing in Vulnerability how he was feeling. He was implicitly telling his audience that he was not different from us. His audience members probably felt anxious prior to public speaking, or maybe avoided it altogether. In that moment he also modeled that fear need not stop us from doing anything. This is a wonderful example of Vulnerability — confronting a fear by turning and facing it, by honestly sharing how he felt and knowing the impact his sharing would have. I sensed his anxiety diminish as he shared this with his audience, allowed the feeling to be without judging it, then let it move through him.

When I am feeling as I feel, it softens and disarms, as I am allowing what is real for me in that moment — firstly to myself and perhaps with others.

How would you like more softness in your life, feeling the strength in allowing self to be soft and tender?

What are you feeling now? Or are you trying to stop feeling by thinking about what you feel?

How would it be to acknowledge what you are feeling without censoring it?

I invite you to feel into how freeing this is and how simply being honest with what we are feeling reduces its intensity as we allow it to be rather than pushing it away.

* * *

Most of us are not taught how to be okay with what we feel and have thus developed many coping strategies to disengage from our feelings. Sometimes we perceive what others around us may be feeling by their projection of it especially if we are empathic as most nurses are. When we judge what we feel, we disconnect from the feeling and either project it out to others or internalize it, pushing it into one of our other bodies, where it doesn't belong, potentially locking it away to manifest in all kinds of ways.

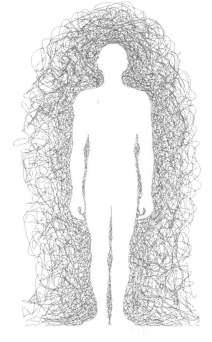

When others are projecting their feelings at us, combined with their judgment of the feeling, it can be an unpleasant experience. Feel into how this is for you. When we deny what we are feeling, we confuse those around us, for they may be sensing the anxiety, but we are denying it.

We can doubt what we perceive as children and take this doubting of self into adulthood, not trusting what we feel. This is why our personal boundaries are so important—so that we do not take on others' energy. Others can choose to be however they like, but we can also choose to engage from a space that preserves our energy field, honoring self and knowing we are of more service to others when we are not being manipulated by the fear in the environment.

How would it be to stop, take a few minutes, next time you are feeling annoyed in your workplace and, without getting caught up in the story, take a few deep breaths and just simply acknowledge how you feel, being grateful for the opportunity, releasing any judgment and choosing the new; perhaps Patience or Acceptance, letting go the old. In doing this, we are taking responsibility for what we feel, knowing no one else can make us feel anything. We can then respond in a calm, more considered way.

We may understand this on a mental level but can easily forget to recall it the next time we are triggered by a person or a situation and move into reaction. We can deepen our commitment to the new by understanding the impact of new choices. Knowing the power in re-choosing or raising the vibration of how we feel in each moment. Simply letting another know what we are feeling and moving away from the trigger to process it can be very effective, as we are not blaming another or denying what we are feeling. This can be disarming to both self and others. We are sharing how it really is for us, taking a chance and sharing that, and then moving away until we are no longer in reaction. Or we may simply withdraw without comment and process our feeling.

When we are expressing a feeling strongly but are not connected to that feeling, it is usually because the feeling is being judged.

Owning our own feelings assists others to own their feelings, and we avoid dumping our unwanted feelings into another's energy field. For example, if I feel anxious but am not aware of this, another person can enter my environment feeling anxious, and I can feel annoyed that I have to deal with this anxious person. If I own that I am feeling anxious, be grateful for noticing and choose Calm Assurance, I am letting it go in this moment and I am not triggered into reaction by another's anxiety. This allows me to protect my own energy field and not project my denied feelings at another. I can then strengthen my boundaries.

This is why telling someone not to worry or to calm down is ineffective, because we are not acknowledging what they are feeling but are, rather, negating what they feel then adding to the intensity by projecting disapproval or by being triggered into our own feelings that we have been denying and suppressing.

As humans, we learn from an early age to protect self from hurt by layering protection around the heart. This is effective at keeping us safe from feeling disapproval and projections of others, but it is not discerning. It also keeps love out, and we can have difficulty letting love in or maybe even recognizing what love is.

Vulnerability is a state of being that allows us to feel as we feel without the need for veils of illusion. It is the honest expression of what we are feeling, and it opens the heart. Surrendering to the knowing of the heart is our natural state of being when we stop rushing and doing. When we are in a state of busyness or urgency and feeling anxious about getting things done, we impart anxiety to all we do, sharing that unease with all around us.

Working with others who are calm and measured tends to have

a calming effect throughout that environment. Feel the difference when you do what needs to be done without the anxiety. We often say we value calm surroundings, but how is each of us contributing to a space of calm? The first step is being honest with self, allowing the anxiety, acknowledging the anxiety is real, being grateful, and judgment can be let go of. Then anxiety can be raised to Calm Assurance or something else, just as all we feel can be transformed into a higher vibration by learning this feeling process.

Raising the vibrational resonance of what we feel can be understood by considering the change of state water undergoes from its densest state of ice to a state of vapor as steam. Ice could represent fear as frozen love; water could be conditional love and steam unconditional love. Changing the frequency at which matter vibrates is possible; all is energy, some in denser forms and some much less so.

The process of raising the vibration of our feelings involves several steps, including allowing, acknowledging, being grateful and releasing any judgment of the feeling. In this chapter, we have explored the value of Vulnerability—allowing our feelings to be, understanding that only when we value what we feel can we access Truth.

Management of our emotions requires responding rather than reacting to others or to situations. We need to become clearer about what triggers us to react. However, much of what has been taught has encouraged suppression of feelings, judging some feelings, such as anger and impatience, to be unacceptable or undesirable. Feelings aren't good or bad but simply are. What we choose to do with the feelings is what impacts us and others.

There is another way to develop mastery of the emotional body—

by allowing the feeling and raising its vibration. This allows us to release the old, which no longer serves us. If we are not allowing ourselves to feel, we are suppressing our feelings in one of our bodies, and if we are storing judged feelings in the emotional body, we can feel anxious and overwhelmed most of the time. Suppression of our feelings can explain those moments when all seems to be going well then—bam!—an emotional outburst as the pressure of suppressed feelings is released, often projected at others. This can lead to self-judgment and guilt and can reinforce beliefs that say change is too hard or faulty beliefs that 'we can't change how we are.'

Emotional maturity is about managing our emotional body, but not by denying or suppressing what we feel.

Many years ago I was working as a Registered Nurse in a general hospital. The morning shifts were particularly busy with many tasks to complete. At the time, I was learning to meditate and doing yoga, seeking a more peaceful inner world, and sought to bring those new skills to my world of work. I would commence the morning shift determined to be measured and calm, knowing I had the skills to do both. However, by morning tea a few hours later, I would be feeling rushed and anxious, like most of the nurses around me, and I wondered how I could create that state of calm I experienced in meditation. I would continue to wonder and go have a cigarette instead, at a loss and disillusioned. I remember feeling frustrated, believing the environment was the problem; but I didn't understand how I was contributing to the anxiety all around. It took me nearly another twenty years to learn. Willing my emotional body to be still was not successful. It was just another way to avoid feeling.

I was yet to learn how to protect my energetic field from the energies of others, and this learning was to have the most profound effect on how I could create a space for myself that was not dependent on the environment I was in.

Hospitals can be challenging environments as we all know. A sea of anxiety pervades all within their walls, and until we have mastered the skill of creating strong boundaries we can absorb that disquietude. The combined anxiety felt by staff around completion of all their tasks and by patients who are unwell and fearful creates a dense energy to which each of us nurses contributes—or we can choose to create something else.

Imagine how it could be if each of us took responsibility for our energy emissions and became part of the solution, creating a different experience where love prevailed, where each of us was able to fully accept ourselves and then truly be there for others?

Chapter 4

Values and Sacred Qualities

If we are not clear what we stand for,
we will stand for anything.
~ Unknown

Being clear on what we value, personally and professionally, helps us master our destiny. I see values as goalposts, assisting us to plot a course in the direction we desire. Discovering our values assists us to know where we begin and what is important to us. Then we can find the gap that can exist where we say we value something but we are really prioritizing something else in our lives. This requires us to raise awareness of what we are feeling, as the heart is where inspiration is found.

There is growing understanding that we do indeed create what we most often think about.

What is your dominant thought?

Let's explore how to create more awareness of what you are thinking.

Some of us may have pretty clear ideas about what behaviors indicate the presence of the espoused values we hold dear and may assume, rightly or wrongly, that others have the same ideas. Others may not have considered what they value, so identifying what is valued is a powerful personal exercise. Then exploring what behaviors indicate which values are displayed or lived by. A powerful and effective way to do this is with a values clarification exercise, firstly for ourselves and then for the teams we work within. This can reduce a great deal of misunderstanding and conflict, as all team members have an opportunity to share their perspective. So much of how we behave can be traced back to the assumptions that others value what we value.

As an example, we can assume that all nurses value the provision of high-quality nursing care and are constantly evaluating their practice to discover better ways of delivering that care. But what if some nurses were more interested in working in a place where people treated each other respectfully? What if those who valued Respect very highly were unable to see how high-quality patient care could be delivered where Respect was not evident for all who worked in that area? If you didn't first explore what you valued within yourself and then within your team, how would you know?

What does Respect look like to you?

We view the world through our own filters and lenses so, until we become conscious and aware of what we value, we often assume it is the same for everyone. Using the example of Respect again: One nurse may believe Respect is shown by valuing each person's contribution. Another may view Respect as something that is directed towards those in authority, assuming they have greater knowledge. Yet another may see Respect as a consideration with which everyone should be treated, knowing they have intrinsic worth and valuing the unique expression each brings. How could it be if all team members were encouraged to share what Respect means to them and how it could be expressed within the team?

How could all team members respect themselves first?

What would communication look like in a team that chooses not only to value Respect but also to display it with the behaviors the team has agreed upon?

This tends to increase accountability of all members of a team.

Until we make our values explicit and look at the behaviors that underpin them, we can be confused, lacking clarity and not be aligned as a team. Rather than just capturing values as words on a page and displaying them, it is more important that we live by them. This can be explored when values such as Honesty,

Trust and Respect—which most people say they value—are unpacked further, bringing to light behaviors that underpin these values. Exploring those underpinning behaviors and looking for incongruence is a vital part of the process. There will often be gaps. The team may agree that they value inclusiveness wherein every team member is valued for her or his unique gifts and contribution, but several members of the team may say they fear sharing their ideas because, when they have done so in the past, other, more senior nurses have told them they were wrong.

Having open, honest conversation takes courage, and each person needs to feel safe in doing this. Teams can then begin to explore the impact of behaviors and decide what changes to try and work towards embracing. Part of the success of this approach requires team members to agree to hold each other accountable to the collectively espoused values.

Team-building days are practiced across many industries. It is recognized that teams communicating clearly will more likely have members who are engaged, contributing, and feeling valued, thus producing a high standard of service. The real work, though, comes after the team-building activity or the values clarification exercise when the team applies the values in their workplace. There is unlikely to be harmony or team cohesion—and, consequently, the team will be functioning well below its potential—until each member has committed to being accountable to the agreed values and to respectfully calling each other on behaviors that may sit outside those values.

Most importantly, before challenging anyone else on their behavior, it is vital we check our own motives and reflect upon what we are contributing to the issue. Sometimes the most 'difficult' team member can have the best ideas as they are comfortable to challenge the status quo; 'the way we do things around here.' Clearing the charge on an issue means to take a breath, acknowledge what we are feeling and not make it about anyone else. Then to release the judgment that we are right and another is wrong. If we do this we can respond to another rather than reacting and they won't feel attacked and defensive. Others will be more likely to listen. Even having the best of intentions, such as wanting what is best for the team, does not guarantee we aren't charged. If we fail to check in and communicate from a place not charged with judgment we project negativity onto another and into our environments. This is disrespectful and contributes to more disharmony. Checking in and clearing the charge means not having an emotional reaction, not believing oneself necessarily to be right. This requires practice and isn't easy after many years of choosing another way but it is possible with persistence, awareness and monitoring.

What is projection? When we communicate with other people we connect by a cord of energy. These cords of energy remain in place until we clear them so take a moment to feel how many cords you may be attached to. As nurses we communicate with others throughout our shift so a considerable amount of energy could have been unconsciously projected at us. No wonder we can feel so drained at the end of a shift. We recall from Chapter 2 that projection happens when we use our energy to feel okay, thrusting our issues onto another. We could also be not owning a behavior within us, judging it as not okay and attributing it to another instead.

Take a deep breath, align, center, affirm that you love the Truth and allow whatever is presenting to be, by asking yourself honestly: What is my part in this situation? What do I need to acknowledge here? Choose Gratitude, and remember to give yourself some time to ponder the questions in your heart, removing yourself from others if possible until you have released any judgment. Re-choose Truth and let go the old. Breathe and Harmonize, feeling displaced energy return to its rightful place.

When I managed a ward several years ago, I knew it was important for me to be aware of what each member of the team valued so that I could understand what motivated them and could match them to roles and activities they enjoyed and that would provide the greatest benefit to the team. I spent time with each individual team member, finding out what she valued, what was important to each person, then asked what she would like to do in the ward that would assist the team to offer the best patient care possible. Most truly wanted the best care for their patients.

However, on reflection, a more effective way of achieving this would have been to do a group values clarification exercise. This was something I would learn down the track. I was a new manager, feeling anxious, believing it was best to build carefully my new relationships with the team, since I was no longer a nurse delivering direct clinical care alongside them. In making this choice which seemed reasonable at the time and was effective, I missed an opportunity for the team to share and understand each other's values and the behaviors that would demonstrate the values being expressed and create a collective set of shared values for the ward. My team also did not get to hear what I valued, and if this is neglected by a manager, the team is left guessing what the manager stands for. I did share my values, but in different moments with different staff members, so it was not explicit for all the team, whereas it could have united us as a team and created a shared vision for the future. When managers share their values with all the team it can be a powerful vehicle for painting a picture of the future, bringing others along on that journey, united in their purpose.

Since working with different groups and teams to create group values, I have heard reports of experiences wherein the team owns the values they have created and feels more purposeful and clear, united in how they will work together. They understand what every other team member requires to do that. When these values are upheld as something each team member stands by, and they have agreed to question each other if behavior is falling outside the espoused value, a mutual Respect is fostered, and assumptions and misunderstandings can diminish considerably.

Generational variants may be present. For example, older team members may value Loyalty more highly than younger members, and younger members may value Adaptability more than older members. Doing a values clarification exercise as a team can be revealing and can create a way forward for a team to write their ideas down and promote flow and synergy. Values are organic and worth revisiting as teams develop. All team members need to feel they have contributed, so new members need to understand how the team arrived at their values and have an opportunity to contribute their own. Displaying the values for all

Kindness	Truth	Curiosity	Hope	Compassion
Adaptability	Courage	Faith	Patience	Understanding
Honesty	Allowance	Surrender	Endurance	Gratitude
Confidence	Unconditional Love	Trust	Appreciation	Sense of Humor
Awakening	Openness	Allowance	Humility	Harmony
Wisdom	Inspiration	Flow	Integrity	Awareness
Worthiness	Calm Assurance	Innocence	Unconditional Love	Loyalty
Clarity of Intention	Clarity of Perception	Receptivity	Connectedness	Unity
Knowing	Mercy	Belief	Realization	Abundance
Charm	Discernment	Oneness	Joy	Purity
Oneness	Serenity	Aspiration	Harmlessness	Attunement
Intuition	Revelation	Is-ness	Illumination	Timelessness

to see is important, but how we engage with those values is where the real worth lies.

We can explore our values in another way: by feeling more deeply rather than just thinking about them. Sacred qualities lie at the essence of all our potential values, both in name and resonance. A sacred quality is a state of being and a quality we embody to live the ideal as humans. There are sixty sacred qualities containing the higher ideals of humanity, each with a unique vibrational key, like a musical note, assisting us to reach constantly for the ideal in the present moment, feeling into its vibration or energy pulsation. Alchemy is simply this: raising the vibration of a substance.

As we live in a duality-based world, we tend to learn by experiencing what not to do. The spectrum of possibilities for learning is vast, so in order to learn to express in the higher bandwidths of the vibration, we need first to experience how we are expressing its lower vibration. We discern where we are not expressing the higher vibration, our barrier to that expression we first need to clear within us. We do this by feeling as we feel without judgment, always in a space of Gratitude, choosing the higher vibration and releasing the old. I often choose a specific quality and explore for a week or two how it plays out within me—loving the Truth and asking myself: How can I express more of the higher vibration?

I have often been surprised while exploring the sacred qualities, sometimes finding that they are not as I had believed. Beliefs are generated from our minds, and sacred qualities are accessed through feeling, so we need a new map to navigate. Feeling into these qualities assists us to experience their essence in a full-bodied way, assisting us to live the ideal of humanity, raising the vibration of our energy fields to ultimately pulsate with all these sacred qualities simultaneously, giving those within our environments an opportunity to experience something other than fear.

When I am facilitating a group, I may sense others feeling unsure of how or what to contribute. In such circumstances, I could feel into the sacred qualities of Hope and Courage, raising the vibration of these qualities within myself and radiating love in the expression of these qualities so that others might feel more empowered to share their knowing. This can also create a space where people feel safe to express in Vulnerability, without pretense. This is possible for all of us to learn and is no longer the secret of a few.

How would it be to learn these ancient teachings?

I will now introduce the seven great Rays to you and how they relate to understanding the sacred qualities. Rays are energies expressed as color and vibration. We can also understand them as attributes or qualities through which light is shared with all creatures on this planet, and we can all access the Rays as we are all aspects of creation. The Rays are seven, just as there are seven primary musical notes and seven major colors. Each Ray has a color and expression unique to it and qualities we can work with to balance and harmonize our expression as spirit in human form. All form structures embody a unique Ray makeup, including this planet and each of us as humans. Each Ray has a lower and higher expression or negative and positive aspect, so we can choose to study the Rays and express through the higher aspects, intending to create more balance and harmony within the self and outside of self.

The beauty of a rainbow splashed across the sky can move us deeply as it is a visual display of the seven great Rays.

We can learn to work with the Rays and sacred qualities together to assist us in our lives. It is beyond the scope of this book to explore the Rays in detail. My purpose in sharing is for you to feel the richness of the unseen world: its interconnectedness and natural order.

Working as part of a team, we may value working together as one, each person playing her or his part to create harmonious relationships with each other for the best patient outcomes. Working with the sacred qualities of Connectedness, Unity and Generosity may assist us to focus our intention on how we may create this.

We may need to have a conversation with a 'challenging' patient or other staff member, so we could call upon Patience and Understanding to assist us with this. Or we may need to complete a task we have decided not to enjoy, so to help us reframe our attitude to this task we could choose Appreciation and Optimism to assist.

With what situation could the sacred quality of Surrender assist you?

How congruent are our behaviors in upholding our espoused values, both as individuals and as members of a team?

How do we address behaviors not congruent to our values?

Nursing has a culture of avoiding critical conversations in which we state our concerns honestly. Instead, we perhaps complain to another nurse and may feel validated, but have we addressed something important to us or simply avoided it? Changing this is crucial to embedding the new paradigm and giving it traction. Empowering every nurse to have the tools to articulate her or his concerns respectfully and with consideration will create teams where everyone feels heard and can contribute.

Allowing ourselves to feel as we feel is an important part of this because until we allow ourselves to feel as we feel, we tend to cast our un-illuminated, denied feelings onto others as energy projections. Repressing what we feel as nurses has a long history. Traditionally, nurses have sacrificed their needs to care for others. This collective history is stored in each of us as nurses and impacts our ability to collectively embrace our professional status.

Ponder for a moment how it could be if each nurse were clear what she or he valued both individually and as team members, and these values were underpinned by congruent behaviors. What if each nurse took responsibility for her or his feelings, allowing the feelings to surface without denying, suppressing or projecting—how this could be?

Can you feel the ease as Flow returns?

Flow is another sacred quality and occurs when we stop banging into obstacles, rather finding a way through, around or over it just as water in a river finds a way.

Let's now consider time and its relationship to experiencing life through the sacred qualities. Time is simply a measure of the flow of consciousness. Consider how we manipulate time every day. When we are enjoying the moment, it passes very quickly; when we are not—perhaps while waiting in a queue, for example—the minutes pass very slowly. Everything on our planet is vibrating, holding an energetic resonance, pulsating at different rates. Our physical bodies are relatively dense, but we can have a very different experience in them if we perceive them as much more than solid bits with basic survival needs running on survival patterns.

Consider how this expanded understanding could alter the fear of not having enough time to do all that needs to be done.

The most important thing is to feel. Feelings are how we access the heart, and through the heart, we access Spirit. We can allow our feelings to be our compass rather than giving the lower mind responsibility for something it was not designed to do.

What if we had forgotten this but now chose to remember?

What are you feeling now?

Sometimes we have done such a good job of denying and suppressing what we feel, we may not even know what we are feeling. We can feel numb. I encourage you to be with your feelings for a moment, quieten the mind, perhaps sensing your mind as a still pool, poised, simply feeling, not having an opinion about what you feel.

Feelings are not good or bad; they are just what they are in this moment.

The repression of feeling is what causes issues for us. The suppression of anger can cause experiences of depression or aggression. When we are truly honest in allowing what we feel, we can raise the vibration as there are no opposites, just degrees, as on a thermometer. We can raise or lower the vibration. Being clear about what we value can assist us to feel as we reflect on what our internal drivers are. Then we can chart our course.

Values or sacred qualities are our signposts, guiding us and assisting us in our lives to make the higher choice, to choose how to live in balance with our values and enhance all aspects of our lives.

Chapter 5

Loving the Truth, Not the Mind

To the mind that is still,
the whole world surrenders.
~ Chuang Tsu

Most of us are taught from an early age to identify self as separate from others, indeed from everything around us. This sets us on a course of believing we have to make it in a world where we are separate from all else. This can be a very lonely place in which to find ourselves, so we tend to form attachments to feel safer, seeking to grasp and hold onto aspects within our environments including people, objects, and even places.

What if we were all One, each an aspect of creation, here to play our parts as unique expressions of creative force and, together, to create the whole? What if our belief in separation were an illusion created by our thinking minds?

The mental body is not just the thinker. It has many levels but for most of us the lower mind runs the show. Placing the lower mind in the captain's seat, allowing it to make decisions is folly as the mind only knows what it has been experienced in this life, thus its knowledge is limited, not tapping into the collective wisdom of the soul that has journeyed through many lives. We place so much importance on the ability to think that we have suppressed our essence, our ability to feel and perceive the world in an entirely different way, drawing on knowledge from a vastness that cannot be accessed by the lower mind.

The lower mind is a powerful tool, able to construct and analyze information in a linear sense, creating boxes to contain all the information it receives and then retrieve it upon demand. Understanding the way it stores so much information helps us understand the origin of our judgments. Giving decision-making authority to the lower mind means every piece of information received needs to be categorized and if it doesn't fit into an existing box a new box needs to be created. To limit the creation of new boxes, slowing the retrieval process, the lower mind makes judgments about group likenesses. This greatly constrains its ability to perceive uniqueness.

Feel into how we are continually looking for similarities to group our experiences and perceptions.

Living our lives by thinking constantly helps us understand the ease in which we judge. It is the design of the lower mind to make sense of the world.

There is another way, but the lower mind cannot show us how. The lower mind was not designed to be in the driver's seat as master of our vehicle, and it makes it a terrible master, never still, flooding our experience with constant thoughts—many useless—seeking to make sense of all the incoming information and placing it into boxes. Our hearts become a distant murmur drowned out in all the noise.

There is growing interest in learning how to think better and this is important in raising our awareness of what we are thinking. It is only then that we can master the lower mind. Most of us are initially surprised at the number of negative thoughts we generate especially against self and how much this inner-critic dynamic limits our potential. Thinking differently can overcome self-defeating thought patterns and foster an understanding of how thinking more positive thoughts of encouragement and upliftment can create a different reality. This is only part of the picture, though, as to live in a full embodied way as intended, we need to perceive inspiration from the heart and make our choices from there, quieting the mind and being guided by our heart's knowing. Then we allow the lower mind to carry out the heart's inspiration.

Using the lower mind as the powerful tool it is, while not being governed by it, requires alert conscious awareness, and this has sparked an interest in the concept of Mindfulness. Mindfulness creates opportunities for us to observe what we are thinking and doing, hence raising our awareness of how many thoughts we have, without pause, tumbling into each other. We are often surprised when we observe our actual experience of this and become aware of how distracting it is and how much energy it takes to constantly think.

Did you know most of us can stay focused on something for only ten seconds?

Beyond Mindfulness is Presentness, which is bringing all our attention here to this 'now' moment and then the next moment so that in each and every moment we are fully present. When we do this our senses are fully engaged. In this heightened state we may hear the birds in the trees outside the window, see the beautiful flower in the garden as we walk by, or see the beauty in the form and subtle hues of the clouds as the sun sets, forever shifting in a constant flow of existence. For many of us, this deeper engagement with our environment happens only when we take a break from work, have a weekend away from our busy worlds. We can, though, experience Presentness in everything we do.

Feel into what surrounds you now that you may not have noticed before.

These experiences provide a richer experience of living and encourage us to feel the connection with all around us. We can choose to engage with life in this deeper sense by simply noticing what is around us.

How could you practice this in your working day?
What could you notice to be more present now?

The late American writer and social commentator, Maya Angelou, was a wonderful example of someone who shared with Wisdom and Humility her experience of Presentness, knowing that this is possible only with constant effort and focus. The desire to be more present is the spark, but it needs fuel to harness that desire, to keep the spark burning bright. The fuel is knowing and being willing to be different; believing in self. Bringing all of self to each moment is possible when we value this more than our mind chatter, allowing the heart to sense and our selves to be governed by its guidance.

Within Presentness is the sacred quality Patience, which is being without expectation. Opportunities present every day for us to choose the best course of action, and to consider from the heart what is the best way forward. Patience allows us to embrace the opportunity without suffocating it in urgency and fear, rather trusting our inner knowing to guide us. The voice of the heart can be very quiet initially as we have not listened so practice and Patience is required.

Our lower minds are of great value, but we needn't allow them to govern all our choices. In losing connection with Spirit, we have given our minds much more to do than they have been designed to do. The lower mind is a powerful tool but not the only tool available to us. We don't use a hammer to tighten a loose screw, but we tend to use our thinking minds to make all our decisions. We have forgotten how many other tools we have available.

Feeling grateful for our lives creates Abundance—another sacred quality—and it assists us to diminish the judgments of the thinking mind. To create Abundance, we must be grateful for where we are now and accept responsibility for what we have already created.

We create our lives in many ways, including the behaviors we choose, the attitudes we hold, the thoughts we have and the words we speak. When we speak our thoughts, they are magnified as energy streams, and we project them out into our environments. Using discernment about which thought we voice and the impact our words have on those around us is one way we can avoid contributing to the mass of negative energy in our environments.

How would it be to practice mindfulness in this way, taking responsibility for all that we speak?

In this fundamental way, we can contribute to the quality of our environments.

Thoughts are powerful energy-forms and, as such, we can make significant changes to ourselves and our environments by raising awareness of what we are thinking and saying and by making different choices—speaking words of upliftment and encouragement.

What is one thing you could choose to do differently today?

Consider the impact this could have in our hospitals, where fear and worry are so commonplace. How would it be if we reduce the heaviness of this experience for everyone and create places of healing, optimizing health and well-being for all? We could create hospitals where people are attracted to work and retain the existing staff as, both individually and collectively, we take responsibility for what is unseen but very much experienced. We can, together, create a very different experience for everyone.

This can bring up resistance; we can justify what we think or say, but Truth is simply Truth, no matter how we try to distort it. What gets in the way of Truth, a sacred quality, is our limited-lens viewing that seeks to justify our own take on what we believe to be true — to make it all about us. Truth is not our interpretation but, rather, what is there when we stand as our authentic selves — without our roles, illusions and glamour. Truth knows no degrees. It is Truth or it is not. Truth can set us free by creating a path to follow out of the dark. It lights the way even if we have only a faint inner sense of what to do next. Trust the heart to lead the way, as the heart, not the mind, leads us to where Truth lies. Trust the heart to lead the way, as the heart is where Truth is sensed. The lower mind knows only this life, whereas the heart recalls all lives, accessing the wisdom of ancient knowing.

Feel for a moment the expansiveness and Clarity of Truth as sensed in the heart. Feel the deeper understanding of the heart. Truth sets us free of limitation, condition, glamour and illusion. With our lower minds, we can be very clever human beings, justifying so many things as being okay when we really know this isn't true. We have instructed our lower minds to keep the truth from us because we fear Truth and its responsibilities. The lower mind is just doing what we have instructed. The trouble is, we have forgotten that the lower mind is simply a tool and not who we are.

What if we could instruct the lower mind to stop filtering the

truth, justifying our behaviors that are less than loving?
How would it be to give the heart back its role, to feel the Truth in each moment and to make choices from that space?

How different could life be if Truth were accessible right now?

Feel into your heart and ask to have revealed an aspect of Truth not previously known.

How might it be if we all lived our lives from this space?

The degree to which we can experience Truth is measured by our commitment to it and our Courage to stop avoiding and denying it, allowing ourselves to feel as we feel without judgment. Yet more than good intentions is required. Good intentions are the starting point, but behavioral change and commitment to that change is what creates that change on the ground.

What in your life is not serving you?

Is it something you know is not in alignment with truth as you sense it?

Feel how your life could be different as you really acknowledge this to self.

How much energy is invested in this denial of what you really want?

How much energy is locked up that could be put to other uses?

How much do you want to free this blocked energy?

Now feel how many other areas could be blocked and how it could be if that energy were freed.

Seeing how much we can avoid and how the mind's inner critic runs its script can release us from the limitation of boxes if we are prepared to be different.

From my own experience a few years back, I had always avoided public speaking as I was very uncomfortable being the focus of attention, but this behavior was limiting me in accomplishing what I felt I really wanted to do—share my passion promoting the success of the graduates of a leadership program I had been coordinating and facilitating. Beneath this fear of public speaking lay a fear of taking responsibility. It felt safer to be small and unnoticed. I had been avoiding shining my light and making a difference in my area of influence. On the day of my first short presentation, I had committed to addressing about 120 people, and I felt anxious. As I stood on the stage and took a deep breath, ready to begin, I realized I could hardly read my notes. They had become a sea of small swirling letters. I had to either feel the fear and do the best I could—speaking from my heart—or step down. In the past, I had allowed fear to be sufficient reason to avoid speaking in public—and countless other things. I decided I wasn't going to be governed by fear and would Trust and draw upon the many tools I had, valuing myself more than the old avoidance pattern I had been running wherein my lower mind said, 'Don't do this', 'You can't do this', 'What do you know?' I felt such a sense of achievement afterwards, not because it was perfect—it wasn't—but because I'd had a go and done the best I could, overcoming another pattern many of us run—'the perfectionist'—which said, 'Don't do anything unless you can do it very well.' This was very limiting and sabotaging as how can we learn new things if we are not prepared to fall short and improve the next time? It is important to uncover how our patterns serve us as this helps us understand why we keep doing things that we so want to change. This pattern had served me, as it had kept me feeling safe and allowed me to avoid taking responsibility and sharing something of value to others.

Can you relate to this or do you have another experience?

What is the inner critic? The voice of the inner critic can be powerful, but only because we have instructed it to be that way. Just as we have created it, we can uncreate it to produce something that will support us in better alignment with our heart's desire.

Much has been written about our shadow side or dark side and the conflict that plays out within us. Many believe this is 'just the way it is', that this duality is part of who we are as human beings. This is not the case. We can heal that which we call the shadow side but not by denying it and pushing it away in shame, judging it as not acceptable. To acknowledge it allows us to see what is there and what fuels it. If we suppress it, we don't get rid of it. We just tuck it away, often shoving it into both our physical and emotional bodies. This can produce physical symptoms and a reactive emotional body that has us feeling overwhelmed and anxious as a default setting. A default setting can mean it seems almost normal for us to be in a state of overwhelm and anxiety. This produces stress on the physical level, which accumulates over years and can cause our organs to break down.

Feel now how this could be different—to simply acknowledge that which you have judged as unacceptable, that part of you so disliked, that you give a hard time to, criticizing yourself.

How does it feel to be with this part of you, giving it space?

We all know how a child denied attention can behave. The child can become louder and more earnest in the desire to be heard and then more energy is required to quieten the demand for attention. This is what we do to ourselves when we deny parts of self, and much energy is required to suppress it. It is important to note that I am not advocating acting on what is discovered but, rather, to simply allow it to be heard. These parts of self that are denied have been created every time we have judged our behavior or judged ourselves to be less-than, or given our power away. Those times when we feel less than someone else or blaming others for our experiences.

How liberating might it be to free up the energy that has been used to deny and suppress?

How might you feel if this energy were available to you?

There is a wonderful old Cherokee story that embodies this message simply and beautifully.

One evening an old man told his grandson about a battle that goes on inside people.

He said, 'My son, the battle is between two wolves inside us all. One is Evil: It is anger, envy, jealousy, sorrow, regret, greed, arrogance, self-pity, guilt, resentment, inferiority, lies, false pride, superiority, and ego.

'The other is Good: It is joy, peace, love, hope, serenity, humility, kindness, benevolence, empathy, generosity, truth, compassion and faith.'

The grandson thought about it for a minute and then asked his grandfather, 'Which wolf wins?'

The old man replied simply, 'The one you feed.'

Our unresolved issues create unpredictable behavior when triggered, and this can derail our best intentions. Our best intentions to change our habitual thoughts and behaviors will be sabotaged by our woundedness and our unconscious fears playing out in all kinds of ways. This helps explain why we sometimes believe we desire a new opportunity and work towards that, then wonder why it seems to fall apart. Or when presented with a new opportunity, we may hesitate, hearing the inner critic saying, 'You can't do that ... You don't have the skills.'

I had this experience a few years ago as an RN working in a mental health setting. As shared in Chapter 3 I was given the opportunity to act as a Nursing Unit Manager (NUM) to cover the appointed NUM's annual leave. Another aspect I considered was feeling reluctant, unsure that I could competently perform the role, and not certain I wanted the responsibility, as I had decided that 'keeping a low profile' was the safest way to be— doing my job to the best of my ability but preferring to be out of the spotlight. This pattern had developed early in my life and had served a purpose, as all patterns do. I believed it kept me safe: I could not be judged and devalued as many managers were. Challenging this pattern created a sense of confusion and Vulnerability and activated all those strategies I had designed to keep me feeling safe.

The process of uncovering the belief system I had created, and had used to justify the pattern, was liberating. I was able to see that the limitation I had been operating under was self-imposed. I began to see that I was free to make different choices and to challenge myself to be more than these patterns and beliefs allowed. I knew on a deeper level, at my core, that I was not learning anything new and that I had more to offer. I was bored and wanted a new challenge, but another part of me was comfortable and wanted to maintain this comfortable status quo. This conflict plays out in many ways until we shine the light and explore those unresolved inner aspects with Courage and Persistence.

I have seen many nurses in a similar space when considering applying for a new position, or deciding not to apply even though they have the requisite skills. New choices can feel threatening. Application of reason from the lower mind to this experience tends to be of limited benefit. Fear will usually flood the four-body system so that we experience discomfort in the physical body, overwhelm in the emotional body, and busy chatter in the mental body, criticizing the new choice as unwise.

Healing begins when we desire to create a different reality and we seize Courage and Determination to open the door and turn on the light. The release found by not holding the door closed frees up energy that has been trapped. This can be a great relief.

Can you feel that possibility of letting go of constraint and limitation that the four-body system endures when we resist going there?

Feel into the possibility of using this newly available energy in new ways as you embrace caring for self at a deep level.

I invite you to take a breath and feel into one of those spaces within, where the light hasn't been for a while, where those judged aspects of yourself that have been denied a voice are hidden. Welcome such an aspect to join you and sit with you a while. Reassure this part of you that you are not judging but are, rather, accepting this unloved aspect and just being with it— breathing and welcoming it, reassuring it that it is safe here. This aspect of you can be placed in your heart when you are ready, knowing that its job is done. Thank it for appearing and being with you, knowing that you are no longer the little child that felt invalidated in that moment. That little child is now safe and loved in your heart.

It is a myth that these unresolved aspects within remain stunted at a certain age. We can heal these aspects, bringing them to our biological age by opening the inner doors behind which they are hidden and welcoming them into the light and back into our hearts.

Most of us have many unresolved, denied aspects within that have been frozen out of our conscious awareness. We may have locked these parts of self away for a long time, denying their existence, judging them as weak, feeling ashamed of them or fearing their vulnerability, so they may not trust us initially. A kind, patient, loving but firm approach works best for parenting our wounded aspects into emotional maturity. Feeling our way is where emotional intelligence lies.

Are you ready to trust the heart to guide you to a new way, allowing your lower mind to take a rest, perhaps seeing it as a still pool, poised?

Chapter 6

The Freedom in Accountability

To be free people, we must first assume total responsibility for ourselves, but in doing so must possess the capacity to reject responsibility that is not truly ours.
~ M. Scott Peck

The concept of accountability may be misunderstood. We tend to perceive it narrowly, to mean what we take responsibility for, like those things that are clearly ours to manage, whether that be our homes, children, patients, pets or upholding any of the many other commitments we have made. Some of us also see it as following through with what we say we will do, being consistent for self and for others.

I see it as all that and much more.

It includes accepting that we create our lives through the choices we make. Sometimes we can accept this on an intellectual level, but other parts of us are not in agreement and this can be playing out in sabotaging ways in our lives. Believing we are at the mercy of fate fuels this belief and can be a common experience for nurses. We live in a free-will universe, meaning we can make whatever choices we like, but we are responsible for the consequences of those choices, always. Accepting this universal truth on all levels of our Being creates a different experience for self and others with whom we engage. It takes a lot of energy to deny universal truth and push up against it with our own limited perceptions — to keep pushing it away.

It requires Courage and a love of Truth to accept and live from this knowing and nurses have no shortage of Courage.

What if the foundation of taking personal responsibility were simply cleaning up the mess we have made—both in a literal sense and at a deeper level of our being? A few of us may have learnt as children to own what we have created, but others not so. How tempting can it be to clean up after others, knowing we can do it quickly and well? This can be a great disservice to those others, whether in our roles as nurses or in any of our interactions with others, as it teaches that there will be someone else to clean up after us and, as we know, beliefs tend to impact all areas of our lives, creating limitation.

One day, I observed a very young child, maybe three years old, in a café. When a woman I assumed to be his mother told him they needed to go, he, without a fuss, picked up the large number of toys he had been playing with and placed them back in a toy box while his mother casually looked on. Some of the toys were bigger than he was and required some effort, but he put them all back, taking several minutes, then scanned the floor making sure he had collected them all. I watched with interest, as what I was seeing was unusual. His mother hadn't told him to pick up the toys nor had she helped him do so. I hadn't seen such a young child or indeed many older children pack up toys without being asked or given assistance. I have often seen toys left scattered over a floor or watched a parent pick them up quickly or a child and parent do it together. What a powerful lesson, to teach children that they are responsible for what they use and it is their responsibility to pack them up afterwards. I wondered how readily this child may approach life, with a firm foundation knowing he can achieve and it takes consistent effort. This left me pondering how much we inadvertently lower the bar for others by building dependence, creating a lack of confidence. What a disservice this is for others.

Clarity about what we are actually responsible for can be revealing, as a common belief among nurses is that we are responsible for everything and we are trained to manage and carry out many tasks in short time frames. It is commonly agreed that the most efficient way to do this is to be a problem solver. Nurses are generous, practical and caring people who want to and do assist others. Fixing problems, whether ours or not, can feel very satisfying. It can affirm our worth and provide evidence of our ability and our status as holders of knowledge and abilities. However, apart from disempowering others, overdoing the fixing of others' problems can leave us feeling scattered and struggling to focus, seeking to discern where we can best make a difference.

The magic of this understanding is that once we are clear about what we are truly responsible for, our sphere of influence expands. Then we can focus our attention and intention where we can directly make a difference, pulling back our energy from the scattered state into a focus that feels clear and full of possibility. This builds momentum, similarly to goal setting. When we make a positive change in one area, it tends to have positive effects in all areas of our lives and we find we have expanded our influence, impacting other areas of our lives.

We live in times where feeling overwhelmed with so much to do is commonplace and nurses particularly struggle with this. Sometimes it feels like a competition for the role of 'who is busiest.'

Simply accepting that there is always much to do and that there will usually be competing demands for our attention can make a profound difference in our lives.

This entails letting go of expectation that it should be different and working with acceptance of 'how it is' rather than pushing against the reality of what is. There are so many opportunities to embrace more of our essence by stretching and growing as we learn more of what we are really capable. We can experience this as overwhelming.

When I explored the belief underlying my own frequent thoughts of having too much to do, I discovered an interesting belief that I shouldn't have to work hard and I should be able to relax, lying supine in a beautiful sunny place, reading and swimming many days in the week! Exposing this belief allowed me to see how I had been creating a situation in which I often felt resentful that I had to work so hard because, back then, I was seeing my relaxation time as an entitlement and felt cheated when it didn't play out that way. Of course we can be unbalanced in our self-care, but this example illustrates the effect our unconscious beliefs can have. Challenging this belief, and choosing to replace it with something more aligned with my priority, released feelings of resentment I had buried, tucked away in different parts of my four-body system.

Now I accept I am choosing to make a positive difference in the world, to contribute more love to a planet that supports and loves us unconditionally, and I choose to assist others to find and live more of their potential. Being clear about what I value assists me to remember and re-focus my energy and brings me back to doing what I can do with a more helpful attitude.

Raising awareness is bringing the unconscious into our consciousness so that we are able to make considered choices based on the direction we choose. Uncovering beliefs and attitudes is a wonderful exercise to do often, as most of us have many of them negatively impacting our lives. Revisiting regularly our beliefs and attitudes is very helpful if we are intent on self-development and transformation of our practice.

Until we uncover our beliefs we continue to reinforce them

unconsciously. I used to often think 'I am so busy'—reinforcing the creation of more of what I know I didn't want: feeling overwhelmed and anxious. Now I choose to have an attitude that is grateful for the opportunities that present themselves, and I know I am a very fine juggler, able to manage many spinning plates concurrently. What if this was the case for you too?

Knowing what drives my behavior and that I can bring more of this into my conscious awareness sustains what I do. I can make new choices and trust my knowing. Keeping a journal is a practical way to assist this exploration. Align to your knowing, center over your heart and ask some self-probing questions like 'How grateful was I today for my experiences?' or 'How much did I empower someone today instead of doing it myself?' Then we need to listen to the answer from the heart. Reviewing our day in this way before sleeping is a powerful tool to uncover challenges and acknowledge growth.

Busyness is also a great distraction from feeling and, often, we will do anything to distract self from feeling, fearing what might be uncovered and how we will manage all those feelings. Resistance to feeling creates much disharmony in our four-body system. The effort of refusing to feel, or judging and pushing away what we feel, is exhausting.

Take a few deep breaths now. Check your alignment, center over your heart. What are you feeling now? Give yourself a few minutes and allow the feeling to surface. Acknowledge that whatever you are feeling is okay. Your feelings are not who you are; they are just there to be felt. Choose gratitude for this oppor-tunity to be with your feelings. Release any judgment of what you are feeling. Re-choose a higher vibration, perhaps choosing the sacred qualities Self-Acceptance or Calm Assurance. Breathe this in as you release the old. Feel the space and stillness you have created as you harmonize throughout your being. Keep breathing.

Can you feel your mind quieter by simply allowing yourself to feel what is presenting?

Let's look at beliefs and how they impact accountability. Beliefs are thoughts we have decided are true and they guide our lives unconsciously until we uncover them. I might believe others are lazy and won't do a good enough job so I need to do everything. Beliefs are not the truth—rather, they are what we have decided is correct. Until we uncover our beliefs we tend to look for proof that our beliefs are correct. So we could attract lazy people into our life to prove we are the only one capable of doing what needs to be done.

Can you see how shining the light on our limiting beliefs could change our experience of life?

Can you feel the possibility of how it could be to uncover what you are actually responsible for rather than what you believe you are responsible for?

What beliefs are surfacing for you to explore?

Many years ago, as a Registered Nurse in a general ward, I used to come home from work after an early shift with good intentions to complete various tasks from the endless lists I created but, often, I found myself in front of the TV feeling tired and indignant, telling myself I deserved to do nothing as I had such a busy day. Then I would fall into bed feeling guilty because I had let myself down. The discarded lists reminded me of my lack of achievement, so I would make more lists that I rarely got to the bottom of. Procrastination is a sign of not being accountable, and I was a master of procrastination, dragging around so much that I needed to do but didn't do or did at the last minute. I cheated myself out of feeling accomplishment, as I often missed deadlines, so I also robbed myself of being able to celebrate success, as I was rushing to the next overdue item demanding my attention. If I had understood personal accountability, I would not have been procrastinating, blaming others and complaining.

Overcoming procrastination also requires an awareness of what we are doing, thinking and saying. Monitoring those thoughts that seek to undo our progress, those thoughts that say, 'I have worked hard enough, done enough and now deserve a rest,' perhaps just as we are close to completing something. When we hear those thoughts we can challenge them and may simple say to ourselves, 'That is not true.' However, if we aren't aware what we are thinking we can't challenge them.

Perhaps we are prone to being overly responsible, believing we need to fix all the issues and perhaps even others around us, as this keeps us from focusing on what is our responsibility. Or perhaps we think what we do is never enough, so we keep doing more, distracting self from what really needs our attention. I have certainly run these thought patterns, and I remember the frustration and exhaustion. Not only did this keep me feeling overwhelmed, it prevented others from discovering what they might be capable of as I was often doing things that weren't my responsibility. As an antidote to this, I now often ask myself, 'How am I enabling others to be responsible and accountable for their lives?' I may ponder further: 'Am I taking that learning from them, disempowering them?' Then I may choose to stop doing that and instead ask an enabling question to assist them in accessing their own innate knowing. Or I may have not noticed I did this until I reviewed my day. It is tough to not give self a hard time about making a mistake but it is really simply an opportunity to improve. Being grateful for the learning helps and

reminding myself to notice next time and make more empowering choices.

Now we will look at patterns of behavior, which are simply
habitual ways we engage with others and situations. It can be
helpful to explore the drivers of our patterns and, for me, several
patterns were contributing to my procrastination behavior,
including 'needing to be needed', doing whatever someone else
prioritized, aiming to please and feel valued. This is a common
pattern that I see in other nurses. We are attracted to a profession
that assists others at their most vulnerable, and knowing we can
make a difference to patients' lives is rewarding. However, when
this pattern is running, we have a need that we are projecting
onto another, so our motive seems to be, 'I am here to assist,' but
can actually be, 'I am here to have my "need to be needed"
fulfilled.'

When this pattern is running, it also means we are not trusting or
accessing our knowing. Instead we are relying on others to
validate us. This also affects how we live our values, as others
may not value the same things we do. We can feel compromised,
as not living in alignment with our values can throw us off
course, leaving us at the mercy of others' opinions or their projections. This can result in feeling disillusioned and not caring that
much. Refusing to take responsibility for my life's direction gave
me the illusion of freedom. I believed that the less I committed to,
the less I needed to take responsibility for. I confused a lack of
discipline with being care free but, in fact, I was unsatisfied and
bored. I didn't recognize or value the gifts I had to share. It is not
possible to identify our unique gifts if we don't first value self.

How much do you value you?
What are your unique gifts?

Exploring patterns that prevented me from achieving success and choosing to take action to heal them allowed me to put something in place to assist my new commitment to self. Had I done this without first exploring the patterns and the beliefs supporting it, I would have continued to sabotage myself in order to validate the unconscious beliefs and patterns I was running. I like to do one thing that I least want to do first thing in the morning—as suggested in a book by Brian Tracy entitled *Eat That Frog*—valuing myself enough to not drag it around for a day, or several days or even months. It is such a relief to get this one thing done, and I acknowledge myself for having completed this task, feeling an ease and flow where achievement is possible for the remainder of the day, opening and expanding the energy flows within.

What is your experience of getting stuck in a pattern and going round and round with it?

What is your experience of completing tasks within deadlines both personally and professionally?

How do you acknowledge completing that deadline before moving on to the next?

Another important understanding that can assist us in becoming accountable and better managing our time is how to live in the present moment. Being present, really present, in each moment means being fully engaged in this moment, bringing all of self to this moment, our feeling, sensing and thinking parts, being in Gratitude and appreciation for what is unfolding. When we choose to relate to each moment in this way we are not overwhelmed, for we are not living in the past or worrying about the future. Allowing one moment at a time, being completely present in that moment, grounded to the earth, connected to something greater than the form density of our humanness by aligning and centering feeling into something much greater, allows us to fully engage with each task, experiencing a 'Flow' state. The experience of being in Flow is possible only when we are fully present in the moment. Recall how, when you have been so absorbed in an activity you loved, hours passed in a moment and you felt at one with the activity. You weren't thinking about it, you were moving with it, whether it was dancing, painting, playing an instrument, playing with a child or animal. This is Flow. If you stopped to think what you were doing, the ease and grace would stop.

Being fully present in each task, whether we have decided it is pleasant or unpleasant, is liberating as it frees up so much energy. It also helps us let go of the judgment of anything being good or bad as really it is us who decide what is good or bad. What we decide is bad says more about us if we are condemning it with judgment. Of course we all need to be clear what we stand for and know where the line in the sand is and what we can do to work for that but it doesn't mean self-righteously judging. Imagine how it would be to not have opinions on everything, replacing judgment with self-acceptance, Compassion and being open to other perspectives. This is how we create more of the culture we want in our hospitals. Otherwise we add to the creation of more of what we say we do not want.

There is perhaps something within accountability that may have extra relevance to nursing if we consider the origins of our profession. Nursing is founded on a transactional management style wherein nurses were expected to have a diverse skill-set but to take all direction from a matron or to be the doctor's handmaiden. Considerable fear and disempowerment were injected into nursing culture, since consequences were severe if orders were not carried out exactly as given. This historical subjugation of female nurses fueled disempowerment and victim consciousness among nurses, and the legacy of that continues to be experienced today. A culture of blame is slowly being put to rest. Risk is now discussed in terms of system failure rather than individual blame. However, what lives on in our nursing collective is sometimes experienced as a culture of blame that permeates throughout all levels of our organizations. Within that old collective there can be a refusal of individuals to take responsibility for the existing culture, expecting someone else to do something about it. Of course management has a part to play in transforming culture, just as each of us has our part to play. Each of us contributes to the culture within our teams, helping to create either teams of empowerment in which each is valued and respected for her uniqueness, knowing a rich diversity produces a culture where everyone flourishes—or maintaining the status quo. Each of us can be part of creating new opportunities or we can be part of that which is past its use-by date and continue to contribute to producing more of the old.

Which part are we choosing to play?

Another interesting question to ask self, and allow time to ponder, is: What effect am I evoking in others?

What am I thinking, saying and feeling? Am I complaining about all that is wrong, or am I uplifting others with a sense of a future that is inspired?

A website named http://qbq.com focuses on this issue of personal accountability, and I found there a very compelling story painting a powerful picture of what this means. A family were traveling home early one evening and noticed a guy climb from his wheelchair and pick up loose newspapers that were scattered across a vacant lot. The family stopped to assist and asked him why he was doing this. He explained he delivered newspapers in the mornings and it wasn't until he'd returned home that he'd noticed a bundle was missing. He then returned to look for the lost papers. Finding them in the vacant lot, he set about picking them up. When one of the family expressed wonder that he would do this, given that he was in a wheelchair, he looked surprised and replied that it was his mess to clean up. This speaks to me about the excuses we can make for not doing as this man did, owning what is our mess and cleaning it up.

How can we apply this to our lives?

Or whose mess are we cleaning up, losing sight of what is truly ours to take responsibility for?

Chapter 7

Being Without Expectation in Our Practice

Your living is determined not so much by what life brings to you
as by the attitude you bring to life,
not so much by what happens to you
as by the way your mind looks at what happens.
~ Kahlil Gibran

Having expectations of how things should be based on what our mind believes is right can seem so normal because we haven't been taught there is another way. Expectations create attachment to an outcome. This limits the myriad ways that exist to create our lives and sets up the see-saw of looking to the past and worrying about the future, keeping us out of the present moment.

When we project expectation onto another, therein lies an assumption that we know the right way for others—but we don't. A simple antidote to expectation is to stop, breathe and choose to feel Grateful for all we have. Gratitude is the key to manifestation so, if we drop into Gratitude we release expectation, opening to the creation of other possibilities. We can feel the stillness and calmness by simply stopping for a moment and breathing. Being led by what we feel in our heart is the best way to find the way forward, acknowledging all the gifts in our lives. When we drop our expectations, self-righteousness falls away and we open to the new, knowing there are always many ways forward when we access creative potential.

Having an attachment to outcomes is a type of expectation and can feel like second nature to nurses. We have been trained to measure our successes as clinicians by the outcomes we achieve, whether they be patients' recovery from illnesses or the brevity of their stays in hospital.

In our roles as nurses, we are most successful when we hold a positive space of Hope for our patients without attachment to their choices. Removing the pressure of expectation from ourselves and others is akin to lifting a weight, because the narrowing of possibility that expectation creates can feel like a heavy imposition. In any moment, a sea of options that we or others may wish to explore is available for our learning, but expectation narrows that range of choices, imposing 'our way' on others, and it may not be the best choice for them as we each have our unique journey, whether in healing or in learning. We don't know the best choice for another, so we can't determine what is best for anyone else. We can, however, uncover our own learning and take that journey.

Nurses can hold a loving space for their patients wherein each patient can explore what is the best option for her in any given moment. This creates a clarity and stillness for contemplation not often experienced in a world intent on giving opinions in the form of advice giving. We are all familiar with providing information to patients for them to make informed choices but it is easy to color that information with what we think they should do. Patients are vulnerable in illness and may feel overwhelmed, looking to us to tell them what to do. Instead of giving advice we can listen allowing them to hear their own thoughts and decide to not have an opinion, simply to listen. This can take practice or perhaps you are already doing this.

How does it feel when we are deeply listened to?

Empowering others to make their choices from a space of love, without expectation, is a wonderful gift to share with our patients and others and is respectful. Respect lies not in assuming we know best but, rather, in seeking to understand, deeply listening.

How do we hold a loving space for others? Firstly, by learning to hold a loving space for self. As nurses, we are caring people, driven by our own motivations and these usually include a desire to assist another in their healing journey. As nurses deliver the care to patients we spend more time with patients than other health professionals. This creates an opportunity to connect with patients, offering something other health professionals can't: the time to connect and build relationships over a shift, the following day and beyond. Mental health nurses understand how the quality of the relationship with a patient directly links to better outcomes for patients. All nurses know this and become frustrated when time is drawn from direct patient care to other activities like data collection. Sometimes in our frustration we can withdraw from the patient, not really connecting and waste the opportunities we do have. Relationships are built on trust and these take time to develop but connection can occur in a minute when we are really present with another person.

* * *

Can you remember a time when you were encouraged to explore without the weight of expectation, when another gave you the space to explore without the need to control the outcome? How did this feel? What did you learn? When patients are ill, a sense of urgency often infuses the environments in which we nurses interact with them and each other, but we can step back and choose Patience, trusting that the patient knows and can access that knowing if we give them the space. Although we may be the holders of some knowledge and expertise, our patients know what is the best choice for them. We can assist others to find their way by asking questions to help build clarity without having an expectation that there is one 'right' answer.

Being without expectation typifies Patience and assists us to not project our energy at others. We often project all kinds of things at others, including our needs. The 'need to be needed' is a common projection of nurses since we are empathic people with a strong desire to assist others. The power of capturing the moment: Role theory can help us to understand this, as the coping role of 'anxious pleaser' is one well known to nurses. Acknowledging and naming what we are thinking, feeling and doing in a moment of difficulty with another can be freeing when we expose that moment, making it easier for us to let go of any judgment we may have of the feeling.

As we have explored, we often judge what we feel, believing that we should not be feeling angry or resentful, for example. We may then choose to explore ways to express ourselves from a role we are developing—for example, 'calm considerate responder'. Being clear about what need is being fulfilled allows us to both understand how the role helps us cope and consider whether there may be another way that could be more effectively diminishing the expectations we have of others. This recognition that we can make a different choice and achieve a different outcome in the next moment is empowering. With conscious intention and persistence we can continue to make consistent changes using techniques that prepare us for known challenges and reviewing events afterwards, acknowledging what went well and what we would like to do differently next time.

We can be acting out our own denied aspects and projecting them onto others then judging those qualities in others as undesirable and annoying. Whatever we judge in another, we may be attempting to avoid or deny within ourselves.

Can you feel into something you judge in another and how that may be within you but judged and suppressed?

How might it be to acknowledge that and feel grateful that

you now know?

I used to struggle with feeling angry, judging it not an acceptable way to feel partly due to some cultural beliefs that females aren't supposed to be angry and partly fearing my own power. Exploring this over a period of time I was able to see that feeling anger was okay as, although it is a feeling that may be powerful, I can choose my behavior in response to any feeling. Suppressing and denying anger was ineffective. I was passively expressing it as sarcasm so that others were still experiencing my anger. Now I support myself in a strong alignment, and I center, allowing myself to feel anger when it presents, owning it, acknowledging it as okay, releasing the judgment and raising its vibration into something else: Acceptance.

* * *

During my nursing training, I lived with a few nurses, one of whom was very compassionate and shared with me how she cared for every patient as if that person were her mother or father. She said this assisted her to provide the best care she could for patients in her care. At the time, I was moved by her sharing and recalled it often in my early nursing career. Now I see that perhaps relating to patients in this way may have projected her unresolved issues with her parents onto the patients she cared for, creating expectations for their progress. This may have limited her ability to greet and be in the present moment with every patient anew, each in his or her own unique expression. She could have instead held a compassionate, loving space for all in her care while not projecting onto them her idea of what recovery may look like.

Professional boundaries can be confusing for nurses. There is a tendency to be either under-involved or over-involved. We sometimes believe that either shutting down or being overly involved are the best ways to cope with our exposure to the suffering of others, but there is another way. Having and maintaining professional boundaries is not about closing down to others. In fact, the opposite is the case as we can care from a space of upliftment and encouragement, allowing others to determine their own futures. Having tools to manage our energy makes this possible.

Acknowledging our feelings allows us to own and manage them, then care for others from a clearer space. When we don't do this, we can be triggered into our own unresolved aspects, drawn into another's story, feeling their experience as if it were our own. Sometimes we misinterpret this as being empathic but it is sympathy. Empathy is possible only when we can get out of our own way and not be triggered into our own experience by what another shares. This understanding illuminates how we can feel so exhausted after a shift as our unresolved issues have been triggered and we have given our energy to a patient so they feel better. The patient may feel better for a short time, but we have disempowered them by energetically agreeing that their situation is indeed terrible and we would not want to be in it ourselves, so we give some of our energy, feeling uncomfortable in their experience. Not being drawn into another's experience in this way can feel uncaring at first but energetically propping up another is disempowering and ineffective for more than a short while. It also depletes and is a leading cause of burnout for nurses. Giving our energy to others every day and not replenishing our own system means exhaustion. Always holding a space of Hope that there is another way allows others to feel encouraged and uplifted in challenging times.

I had a powerful learning with this many years ago when, as a twenty-year-old nursing student on a placement in a children's oncology ward, I was allocated the care of a three-year-old girl.

Her mother was not much older than I and had another young child at home with her husband. I kept wondering how this mother could handle this and remain so positive? I felt like crying every time I spoke with her as her little girl was very unwell. The mother would get up at 5.30 each morning, dress, and present herself to the world smiling and feeling grateful for the time she had with her seriously ill daughter. She would share with me her gratitude for all her many other blessings: her loving husband, the health of her other child, the quality of health care available, the caring nurses ... and her list went on. She taught me much during my eight-week placement about the importance of a positive attitude and of not judging what we are presented with in life. We spoke often, and I felt many confusing feelings during and after our conversations. At the time, she struck me as unusual, as she was generous and warm, felt deeply, expressed what she was feeling without inhibition and embodied such strength. She was holding a space of Love and Hope, not only for her sick child but for all of us in that ward, not allowing us to treat her as a victim but, rather, as a woman blessed with an opportunity to develop Compassion, resiliency and Courage to keep going, living from this Now moment. She seemed to have no expectations for her daughter, and she didn't burden her with the weight of wanting her to be anything other than what she was, instead cherishing the time they had together. Her daughter was relaxed and calm, secure in her mother's love that was not conditional on her recovery. She took great care that the relationship was not centered on her daughter's illness, and they played, laughed and talked. Sometimes they cried together. I didn't know it at the time but this young woman showed me a window into my future as I could go on and teach others what she taught me.

Being without expectation is respecting another's right to choose her way, not imposing our way assuming we know what is best.

Seeking permission before we share is one way to check whether another seeks our input and whether the time we choose is right for that person also.

I invite you to feel how it feels when another offers you advice, which often begins with 'You should ...'
Are we receptive?
Do we feel imposed upon?
Do we feel respected?

Sometimes patients can seek advice from everyone as they are frightened, not trusting their innate knowing, believing everyone knows better than they do. This could be an imbalance, and we may be dishonoring that patient by giving advice. Empowering others is learning to ask questions that invite exploration. Others can then be assisted to access their knowing. Empowering patients to be responsible for their health is being person-centered and this approach offers a richer, more satisfying way of working for all nurses, as we become companions on the healing journey.

Holding a loving space for another is very empowering because we don't have expectations for them or judge their choices; rather, our energy holds the qualities of Patience and Acceptance, allowing for accessing a deeper knowing. This space feels encouraging, expansive and full of possibility since we don't assume we know best or impose on another. We allow others to take responsibility for self and we take responsibility for self.

Being non-judgmental is a dictum with which we nurses are all familiar, especially if our background is in Mental Health Nursing. But what does judgment really mean, and how do we know when we are judging? A more revealing question might be: When aren't we judging? Judging is deciding something is good or bad, right or wrong. Most of us constantly judge self, others and all around us. Judgment is a mental activity that keeps us from feeling by repressing what we don't want to see. Judgment also keeps us from the Truth. Remember, the Truth just is no matter how we rail against it, wanting it to be different from what it is, and the Truth can only be accessed from the heart by feeling. Since judgment is a mental activity, it opposes opening to the Truth.

Judgment locks up energy. It contracts and seeks to control. We can learn to release the judgment of self and others and experience freeing up more energy as we learn to flow with life instead of pushing up against obstacles. We can find another way. Gratitude is the key to releasing judgment because we cannot judge when we are in Gratitude, true Gratitude. Gratitude opens us to the possibilities that present constantly, encouraging us to try another way. Gratitude expands and ripples out in our lives, finding the gift in every moment.

Engaging with others without judgment means we can remain in our Integrity and not get pulled into another's story. We can be in Compassion, holding a loving space. We assist others by being without an opinion, allowing others to find their own way and knowing they can change their situation if they choose.

How might it be to not have to have an opinion on everything?

Being without judgment doesn't mean not taking action in what we stand for. It is important to be clear about what we do stand for so that we can create more of it. As discussed in Chapter 4 on values or sacred qualities, there is a difference between moving away from what we don't want and moving towards what we do want. It is much more effective, energetically, to be passionately for something and moving towards it rather than against something and moving away from it, creating a polarizing effect. We experience the notion of opposites when our minds interpret differences through judgment. We can experience this in another way when we notice that energy vibrates at a higher or lower frequency, and we can contribute our energy to that higher frequency. This is why goal setting is so effective: It challenges us to be very clear where we are heading, what it is we are giving our energy to and to monitor our progress.

Gratitude shifts our perspective. We can thus acknowledge all that presents as an opportunity to learn rather than to control our experiences. We can allow Gratitude to guide us in and through life. Without expectation, we cannot be disappointed by others' behavior or our own. We embrace the learning and know we will have another opportunity.

Life is an endless stream of opportunities, and we choose what we will do with each one as it presents. The more we can live in the moment, the Now, the more likely we are to notice the opportunity that is presenting and make a conscious choice how we will respond to it. Even Gratitude is a choice.

What are you choosing now?

Are you feeling grateful for your life? All aspects of your life?

What could you feel more grateful for?

An effective tool is honestly reviewing each day, from an aligned and centered space, affirming that we love the Truth, asking how much gratitude we were in and reviewing again at week's end to know if more gratitude has been chosen. This raises awareness of what we do and the results we get—very simple and highly effective. We can then move towards, rather than away from what we don't want, continuously assessing how we are achieving what we value by expanding our awareness, reviewing what we do, think and speak, one step at a time. Learning to ask ourselves questions that access deeper parts of self can be very revealing. In order to install new behaviors, we can make use of a visualization tool employed by sportspeople for many years now. Make some time each day, always from an aligned and centered space, and take five minutes, using all your senses, to see, hear, feel, touch and taste what you want to create. This engages our unconscious mind, which doesn't work linearly so doesn't need the actual experience to believe it has occurred. This is how visualization techniques work—by reinforcing the 'lived' experience of the desired outcome. This technique is highly effective for many across a diverse range of occupations, and doing this from an aligned and centered space makes it even more effective.

Listening to the voice of the heart, we are encouraged to be more of who we really are. Challenging our self-imposed ways of limitation is not the easiest path. The path of most resistance calls us to achieve more than we may have believed possible, knowing we are and can be so much more. The heart continuously challenges us to stretch and develop—to live a life of continuous learning, exploring new ways of being in the world, being in Gratitude, taking responsibility for the life we have created. As we do this, we encourage and give permission to others to do the same, modeling new ways of Being without expectation.

Chapter 8

Limited-Lens Viewing

Love recognizes no barriers. It jumps hurdles, leaps fences, penetrates walls to arrive at its destination full of hope.
~ Maya Angelou

We are created to learn, growing and developing to be more of our true nature as we live each life, increasing our understanding and compassion for self and others. This requires discipline. As this is a choice, we can choose not to grow in understanding and compassion, getting stuck in the limited-lens viewing we tend to create as young children in order to cope.

Our worldview or attitude towards life develops when we are very young, and this creates our frame of reference—the lens through which we view life. We can remain stuck, experiencing life from this perspective and assuming others have the same view of reality. I know I have done this at many points in my life. Assumptions are the cause of much conflict on this planet because our assumptions about life can remain hidden while we use them to navigate our way through life. Expanding our worldview requires giving up our narrow perspective, and this is uncomfortable. Sometimes we can value feeling comfortable quite highly and resist challenging ourselves. Or we may see what is required but refuse to change our behavior, deciding we are not ready or we are not willing to give up what we know.

Our attitude toward life ripples through all we see, think and do, impacting all it touches. We can be unaware of how much limitation we are placing on ourselves because we form these attitudes so early in life, before the age of seven, and they operate through our unconscious minds, influencing all we do.

As a young woman, I came across a study of a group of ordinary suburban kids in a documentary series called *Seven Up*, which explored these themes. Australian film director Gillian Armstrong gathered a group of seven-year-old children in Adelaide in the early 1970s with the intention of returning every seven years to capture their lives again, asking them the same questions about their lives, attitudes and beliefs. Some of the original participants chose not to continue in the study as their lives had not lived up to all they had hoped for. One developed a mental illness and was living alone in a caravan in an isolated part of England. *Forty-Nine Up*, the latest installment, is fascinating and challenging viewing, as the lives of these people mirror our own. Some have retained the positive attitudes of their younger selves; others have re-evaluated their attitudes and created something else. Others weren't expecting much from life and they struggled to create a desired life. As an audience we are privy to how the attitudes these adults held as seven-year-olds can continue to inform their lives so many years later. I am grateful to these people who courageously shared their lives with us helping us to explore what our responses might have been, had we been asked at seven-year intervals how we were living life.

Attitudes we don't explore and challenge keep us stuck in the past, operating from outdated ways of being and preventing us from taking advantage of new possibilities that present in our lives, or even sabotage our efforts to achieve in all areas of our life. We form an understanding of our experiences based on perceptions and judgments we formed as young children then attribute meaning to them. This is the limited lens through which we evaluate life.

Consider for a moment a group of people who have experienced the same situation with each attributing a different meaning to it. So what we attribute meaning to often says more about the viewer than the event. Exploring the meaning we have attributed to different events is a powerful way to bring to light these buried treasures.

Did you know that police rate eyewitness accounts as the most unreliable for this very reason?

We all see something different according to what lens we are viewing the world from.

Just as we regularly review our patients' responses to our care and treatment, we can review our own attitudes, widen the lens through which we view life, and decide what is helping us and what is hindering us.

Consider what thoughts you habitually think and some favorite ways of expressing them to reveal deeper attitudes of which you may not be consciously aware.

We choose our attitudes at a young age to make ourselves feel safe, so these are coping mechanisms we put into place to cover up the truth of our experiences. This provides a layer or filter that allows us to feel better about an aspect of life that challenges or threatens us. The attitude once served a purpose, but what purpose does it serve now?

As a young girl, I decided the world was an uncertain place and that others couldn't be trusted, so I set about being very independent and not needing anyone. This independence was created from a sense of fear, though, and I constantly tested my belief to reinforce its validity, proving that most people were unpredictable and could not, indeed, be trusted. Validating my beliefs was a great survival program, and I was able to keep others at arm's length where they could not harm me.

Several years ago, I decided this attitude and lens of the world no longer served me and I set out upon the journey of discovery. I continue to learn how I create my future with my thoughts, beliefs, values and expressions. I decided I no longer wanted to live my life acting like I was separate from all else and experiencing life as a victim. I set about monitoring my thoughts, attitudes and most importantly getting in touch with those feelings I had suppressed. This is a choice we all have, and it shines a light on how some people who have experienced much suffering in their lives can remain positive and compassionate as they maintain Hope beyond the moment by refusing to relate to life as a victim. This doesn't mean it is easy. No one's life is easy. Life is challenging and an unfolding process that continues, but if I can do it, it is possible for us all.

Choosing to monitor our thoughts, attitudes and feel what we are feeling allows us to raise awareness of how we are operating in the world, identifying what we can do differently. Setting our intention to notice what we are thinking and speaking and allowing our feelings keeps this in our present awareness and, each time we take note of something we think, say or feel, that enhanced awareness supports us in creating even more awareness, an ever expanding awareness. When we notice something that doesn't support what we value, we can stop, take a breath, affirm our connection and alignment to what we do value, center in the heart, feel Gratitude for noticing, let go any judgment of self or others, and choose our new way, letting go of the old, allowing harmony to radiate through our being.

In Chapter 7, we explored Being without expectation and gained an understanding of the gift we give to others when we don't routinely offer our opinions. Our opinions are formed from our own biases and filters so, until we become more consciously aware of what they are, we are sharing from only a narrow bandwidth of understanding or our limited lens. This also limits the possibility for others to access their own knowing. If we can hold a space of unconditional positive regard for another, no matter what the relationship, the other feels valued as we are fully present and free of judgment for whatever they share.

Have you had an experience where another has held this space for you?

How would it be if you held this space for self?

In order to hold this space for others you must first do so for self.

To be without judgment, we need to be aware where our beliefs and biases lie and have a desire to look and courageously face them. Recognition is the first step, followed by the healing of those wounded aspects within. Until we heal those aspects, those hidden parts of our selves can be activated without warning, and we can find ourselves in emotional reaction. The importance of psychological clarity cannot be overestimated. Our degree of conscious awareness is limited, and we can heal only that which we are prepared to face and bring into our consciousness. Standing and facing what most frightens us. I love this expression by Jung:

One does not become enlightened by imagining figures of light but by making the darkness conscious.

Conscious awareness is the alignment of what we say we want with our actions. We all carry un-illuminated aspects within and, when those aspects are triggered, it often results in 'unpre-dictable' behavior. We may wonder where that reaction came from and why it was so strong when the presenting issue may appear to be quite mild. As we go about our lives, we bump up against each other's denied aspects often and can feel dismayed at some of the reactions from both ourselves and others. It takes courage to face our own shadow aspects. We can see others' denied aspects more clearly than our own as they mirror those parts we deny in ourselves and judge as unacceptable.

An example of this occurred for me a few years ago when I was asked to deliver a session in a workshop that another facilitator was planning. I felt she didn't value my work, based on some earlier interactions. I was initially surprised, wondering why she had asked me to deliver a session. As our discussion continued she challenged the value of my contribution, and I felt threatened, angry and defensive. To avoid responding in anger I retreated and felt into the mirror she presented to how I devalued myself, not acknowledging what I had to share. Others' opinions about us cannot affect us if we value self.

I was also judging the other person, feeling angry. Removing ourselves when we are triggered, rather than reacting, is useful so that we can process what we are feeling and not project this onto another. It may be helpful to inform the other person that you can't talk now but will talk later when you have processed and can own your own reaction. You may eventually accept that you have responded in this way because you have unresolved aspects—feeling 'not good enough' as in my case—and this aspect has been triggered.

If I had denied this, I would have continued to blame the other for not treating me properly and would have continued to feel angry with her. Instead I recognized the intensity of the feeling aroused and, rather than projecting it onto another, I felt grateful to be shown this part of self that I had judged and denied and, by acknowledging it, I was able to transform the experience into something else, enabling me to heal on a deeper level. This is what we call bringing back to self what we feel about another. It doesn't mean we don't take a stand for ethics and integrity but knowing we are more effective when we come from a place less clouded with our unresolved issues. We also value self enough by having strong personal boundaries based on love for self and others, not allowing others' projections to enter our energy field.

To be without judgment is possible only when we become more aware of what we feel, releasing judgment and choosing a higher vibration of the feeling—doing this for ourselves first then inspiring others by modeling another way. We can allow others to make their choices. Not imposing what we believe may be best. This can be challenging in nursing where many of us are in the roles of 'frustrated fixer' or 'anxious pleaser.' These coping roles serve us if we are okay with feeling frustrated or anxious, but how would it be to experience something else?

I have had the privilege over the last few years of assisting clinicians as both a coach and a reflective clinical supervisor, walking beside other health professionals to help them find new ways of being in their clinical practice. Traditionally, the nursing profession hasn't valued reflection as important. When I trained in the late 1980s we were trained to be skilled problem solvers valued for assessing and making quick and accurate clinical decisions and deciding when to seek further advice. Then there was always another patient to attend to, so we promptly moved on to the next issue at hand. We were trained to have a 'chin up' approach to less-than-desirable outcomes, and we carried these painful experiences with us by just tucking them away. Support was not deemed necessary. This was just part of being a nurse.

Sometimes you might be asked, 'Are you okay?' with the expectation that you should reply, 'Yes.' Nurses who trained in the hospital system have all shared similar experiences when I've talked with them, and many welcome another way to make sense of our practice. Of course, some nurses would reflect on their practice but it would tend to be from their own volition or inherent reflective natures. I was naturally reflective, but being reflective doesn't mean I did anything differently as a result of those reflections. I would ponder and observe what I felt but would not often take different action to get a different result. Reflection on its own can be passive and not productive of change, and I understood this well.

I was delighted to be exposed to Action Learning Sets in 2008 when I completed a leadership program in my area health service. I was able to apply my reflections on and in nursing care and make behavioral changes and could assist others to do likewise. Action Learning Sets are a structured process in which a closed group of four to six people commit, usually for a limited time, with the intention of assisting the presenting person to reflect on a work-based issue and discover a new way forward. The group builds trust and rapport prior to commencing this activity and endeavors to be both supportive and challenging with enabling questions. The group usually meets monthly, and the process ends when the presenter of the issue decides on one or more actions to try, then feeds back to the group, sharing how their actions worked prior to implementing the next set the following month. Each group member has the opportunity to be a presenter. Advice is not given to the presenter. Each presenter is deemed the expert in their context and knows at their core the way forward. Instead we assist the presenter to access their knowing with coaching techniques and, most importantly, a safe, attentive, non-judgmental space.

The sense of delight, or the 'ah-ha' moment recognizing that there is another way and it has been accessed within, is very empowering and can be a revelation to many. Having the full attention of a small group of people was a gift to the presenter as the focus is on assisting the presenter to find a way forward. Feeling lighter is a common experience after a session, whether it be coaching or an Action Learning Set, as new possibilities have been found. When we can't find our own way forward we feel stuck and can believe there is no way forward. Conscious behavioral change is the only way the new can be integrated into our lives, and this can be the next challenge—for people to maintain awareness of the new behavior and make it achievable—as small changes done consistently are most successful.

Working with people in reflective practice—coaching, doing reflective clinical supervision, mentoring or delivering workshops—shows me how much limitation we can place on self with our belief systems holding us in check. Challenging assumptions is an effective coaching technique because we all tend to form our understandings based on assumptions we have made, and these are often focused around others' behaviors. A simple example may be that I might assume my manager is not interested in my ideas because when I knocked on her door, she sounded annoyed and said she couldn't talk as she was busy. I could retreat and not seek to approach her again, feeling rejected and unappreciated, when the truth is that she was simply busy and would be interested in hearing my ideas at another time. This scenario may seem obvious, but serves as an example of how, when we believe we are not valued, we are easily hurt by others. We tend to judge others as it is a big deal for our emotional bodies. I could refuse to feel these feelings of rejection and unworthiness and miss an opportunity to explore what was really happening. It is only when we are able to step back from what we are engaged with, to feel how we feel, that we may see another perspective that wasn't initially apparent.

We create our belief systems to keep us safe, so we tell self that certain situations are dangerous and to be avoided at all costs, so that we will not do it again—whether that be opening to intimacy with another or exploring the bush or a myriad of other possibilities. Beliefs tend to develop when we are young and dependent on our parents for survival, so we tend to take on their beliefs until we evaluate them and possibly choose to disregard them as not appropriate to how we choose to live now. The importance of bringing these beliefs into our conscious awareness may be best understood by feeling into the knowing: We can change only that of which we are aware, so making the unconscious conscious is the key.

Another way to raise awareness of our behavior and the impact it has on others is to ask. We can request feedback from others, both formally and informally. We may have blind spots of which we are unaware where others see a behavior that limits us. 360% feedback is a useful formal tool for gathering richer data: a range of people we value, including our managers, peers, people we manage (if any) and others are asked to give feedback, both qualitative and quantitative. The data are then analyzed to produce detailed visual representations and used to help us to see our blind spots and to acknowledge hidden strengths.

Being open to receiving feedback is important, but we always need to be in our discernment, as we are only able to offer feedback through our own filters and lenses, and if we are receiving the feedback, we can make sense of it only through our filters and lenses. Choosing our language carefully is important. Many of us run an 'inner critic' program that judges self harshly. The inner critic dynamic constantly scans our environment looking for evidence of our dysfunction, and we criticize ourselves more harshly than the external world does in a belief that external criticism will be less painful if our own is harsher.

The degree of clarity or awareness we have assists us to give useful feedback to others and also to be receptive to it. An example may be if I am giving feedback to someone who avoids confrontation while I have a belief running within me that it is unsafe to raise my concerns and, if I am not aware of it, I can project my desire to avoid, blame the other party, and keep the other in limitation. Or I can feel angry that the person to whom I am giving feedback isn't dealing with her issue and may project my judgment onto her, leaving her feeling judged, hopeless, and generally more disempowered. There is a great deal of responsibility to giving feedback so being in a clear state is important.

Maybe I have a belief that acknowledging anger is unacceptable, so I could feel intense aversion towards another who displayed their anger, as they are holding a mirror to my own denied anger. In this way, we are all mirrors for each other, and we can sense the challenge in communication when each of us is running patterns of behavior and beliefs that we deny and others mirror them to us.

The most empowering way forward is to discover the Truth within by desiring to know the Truth and calling forth the Courage to be honest with self, trusting the heart to lead us towards making different choices based on love and harmony and on knowing this is possible for us all. We are all aspects of creation in various stages of uncovering that jewel that resides within each of us.

Martin Seligman, in his book *Authentic Happiness*, emphasizes that focusing on the problem and how to fix it should not be our priority. Rather, time should be spent enhancing the positive parts of self, using our strengths to grow our weaker areas. This may assist our understanding of lens as he encourages us to take a positive approach. We all know we should be positive in our approach to life but finding how challenges us. Knowing we can open the limited lens we may be viewing life from and see through an expanded self-loving lens offers another approach.

Really, possibilities are endless.
It is our minds that create limit.

Listening to the heart is where the new exists.

Chapter 9

Embracing Courage and Endurance to Overcome Resistance

You cannot discover new oceans without the courage to lose sight of the shore.
~ André Gide

The sacred quality Courage is fundamental to all of us on this planet. Without Courage, we could not progress as humans, moving with Spirit through the relative density of the human form. These timeless, sacred qualities assist us at a core level on the path of self-improvement as we journey through life, uncovering our potential. Without Courage, we succumb to fear—fear of the unknown, fear of change, fear of success, fear of failure. A commonly held belief is that we fear failure, but many of us fear success and the responsibility success brings.

As I grew up in the sixties in suburban Melbourne, the sacred quality of Endurance didn't seem important to those around me. I don't recall anyone around me displaying much of it. Of course this memory is seen through my personal lens and the filters I viewed life through. Life back then seemed easygoing for most, and egalitarianism seemed pervasive in my world. All of the families I knew were single-income: fathers as the breadwinner and mothers home before and after school. This apparent even playing field created a neighborhood where lives seemed to be lived simply and without too much fuss. Although kids were encouraged to do well at school or in sport, Endurance wasn't encouraged as something really necessary for success. It was almost as if displaying Endurance would have been seen as unbalanced, as working too hard. Downtime was encouraged for kids and adults alike, to play and enjoy life. Work was work and play was play and there didn't seem to be much crossover. Although this assisted me to appreciate a work/life balance and I am grateful for those simpler times gone by, I wondered how it would be to love what you did and not see work as something that was just necessary to earn an income or an education. This possibility was something rare, I was told, and only for those with special gifts that were apparent at an early age. I didn't appear to have a special gift so, with little self-determination or Endurance, I set aside for many years the idea that I had anything much to offer.

Endurance is not giving up when the going gets rough. It is finding another way when barriers present. It is knowing we are worth giving it our best shot.

What was your early experience of Endurance?

How do we measure the presence of Courage in our lives?

Do we look for grand expressions of Courage in others and measure ourselves as lacking in comparison?

Or do we acknowledge when we feel fear but courageously still choose to step up to a new challenge with Endurance?

The quality of Courage is so important on the path of self-development, as there will always be many reasons why the new doesn't seem possible. Finding the compelling reason to take that next step anyway and taking action to move forward in that direction often requires a great deal of Courage, especially if we have been stuck in inertia or sitting comfortably in doing something well for a while. Taking the first step creates some momentum for the change, creating movement out of the inertia then, like a wheel that has started to turn, change is set in motion and a new path opens; we can then choose to maintain the momentum.

Fearing the unknown and doubting our abilities can be parts of a survival program our subconscious is running, but just as we have chosen to run this program, we can also choose to discard it. That can be as simple as consistently choosing another way, a more loving way, and remembering our new choice as the moments unfold before us. We can make all this much more complicated than it is but it really is very simple. Only when we understand and cultivate an awareness that we are much more than a series of programs can we draw upon deeper reserves of empowerment.

Who do you believe yourself to be?

How is Courage displayed in your life?

How much do you value Courage as a quality that can assist you toward your best expression of Self?

Give yourself time to be with these questions, affirming you love the Truth.

Truth is another sacred quality that is foundational to self-development. Breathe and ponder in your heart. Self-questioning can be very empowering because we are effectively being our own coaches uncovering our patterns of behavior and the blocks we have placed in our paths. Be open to the Truth that lies at our core. This is a dormant part of us lying deep within, waiting to be awakened, and it reminds us we are part of something much more than what we think.

Without significant amounts of Courage, it is not possible to achieve our goals. Courage seems to be a quality that a few embody in all aspects of their lives. We may sense that Courage is lacking in our lives, but this may also be deceptive, as Courage may be demonstrated but not recognized in some aspect of our life, and this Courage can be drawn upon and transferred into other areas.

Take another breath and feel into each question.
Where do you exhibit Courage?
Where would you like to exhibit more of it?
What motivation underlies this Courage?

When our motivation is for the greater good, we can harness this energy, as history has illustrated time and time again. How can we check whether our motivation is selfish or selfless? Have the Courage to honestly reflect who or what will benefit from our acts of Courage, always affirming that we love the Truth and courageously plot our course to serve the greater good.

Now we will explore how goal setting can assist us to overcome resistance.

What has been your experience of setting goals?

Working with people for the last few years in assisting them to create goals has shown me the resistance many have to capturing their goals. Writing them down means a commitment has been made. This was certainly my first experience of creating goals. I found it challenging and I avoided writing anything down for some time. I wasn't sure what I wanted to achieve. I just knew I wanted life to be another way. I persisted in a kind but firm way with self and created small steps. A common barrier most of us place in front of ourselves when goal setting is making the steps too large and the time-frames too short or non-existent. Goals need to be SMART: specific, measurable, achievable, realistic and time-framed.

I was inspired by this simple line: 'A goal not written is just a wish.'

In Chapter 4 we explored our values and our values can greatly help us to frame our goals as being clear about what we value forms the foundation for creating meaningful goals.

Dividing goals into four parts can also assist: professional, personal, health and spiritual are useful places to start.

Would you like to have a go at goal setting now?

I encourage you to take colored pens or pencils and paper (at least A4 size) and divide it into four parts with the above suggested headings and take a breath, align, center and ask your higher knowing to share with you what you desire to achieve. Write or draw whatever comes to you, not censoring, just allowing and letting it flow. See this as a heart-storming exercise. Take a good thirty uninterrupted minutes to do this—no calls, Facebook or snack breaks; just you and your heart's desire.

How did you do with that exercise?

It can be challenging. Maybe we haven't considered what we really want and how we will achieve it, or maybe we have become aware that one part is well planned but not another.

On which part would you like to place more focus?

Take another deep breath, a fresh piece of paper and heart-storm what you would like to achieve in that area of focus—not how you will get there, just what you would like—using all your abilities to really sense and create this. Take at least ten minutes to ponder and capture your ideas. Now circle which one you will act on first and apply the SMART framework. It is important that a goal is specific, measurable, achievable, realistic and time-framed so that we know we have achieved it. Now the fun part: You get to break this down into steps. An example of a goal might be: I value my health and will swim three times a week to improve my fitness so that I can climb three flights of stairs and breathe easily. The actions might be to check out local pools tomorrow, buy swimming costume, cap and goggles next payday, join pool of choice on a nominated day, swim after work on Tuesdays, Thursdays and Saturdays at 4pm, and climb three flights of stairs at least weekly and record ease of breathing.

Now that you have created a goal, set some actions for achieving it so you can monitor your success and celebrate the gains. It is commonly accepted that it takes 28 days, or a full lunar cycle, to create new habits of behavior, then the new neural pathways have been formed and the new behavior integrated. A common slipping point is the last week of implementing new behavior, so this is when it pays to acknowledge the benefits of our new choices and choose to work with the sacred quality of Perseverance to follow through and achieve our goals. Goals stick when we imbed small changes every day, bringing the new to fruition. Acknowledging your success to sustain your commitment to the new.

Goal setting can be fun and is simple.

Nurses have great organizational skills so once we get over the resistance we make great goal setters.

Let's have a look at how we can maintain our values in the teams we work within and how Courage and Endurance plays a part. Being clear whether we are still on track, heading in the direction of our values, and whether our values are in alignment with the organizational values in which we operate means it is valuable to review this often. The most challenging part for all of us is to identify how our behaviors express what we say we value. Often, we will find a disconnect between what we say we value and what our behaviors say, reminding us of the saying: 'Actions speak louder than words.' Most of us can recognize others' behavior that falls short of our values, but can we own our own behavior? We can courageously choose to look at those behaviors that are not in alignment with our values and make a new choice one moment at a time. You may now be experiencing a deeper understanding of the importance of loving the Truth as without the Truth we have illusion and denial but can convince ourselves we are doing just fine.

We may, for example, believe we value the quality of Respect for others, but we may have been excluding some of the other nurses at work because we don't see them as competent nurses, able to complete the tasks for which they are responsible.

How do we manage this in a new way when our hospitals are so very busy and are often understaffed?

How do we express Honesty that has universal appeal?

How prepared are we to have honest communication with others, while being respectful in how we do this?

How prepared are we to ask what others are experiencing before we voice our discontent with them?

As a profession it is challenging for nurses to have open and honest communications with each other but I know this can change, one conversation at a time, as more nurses become empowered; owning their value and contribution.

There is a culture of busyness in our hospitals and indeed across many aspects of our lives, where 'success' can be measured by how busy we are. Busyness is 'doing in urgency' and creates anxiety; and anxiety is contagious, especially without strong personal boundaries. We may believe that if we get all those tasks done, we will feel relieved; but are all the tasks at work ever completed? At home? This then fuels the cycle of busyness. We have never ending lists of tasks to complete and seem stuck in the cycle of being busy, believing this is the only way we can get it all done.

What if we accepted that there will always be much to do but we can choose how we complete the tasks?

Choosing to complete them from a space of calm attentiveness, without the urgency, could be another choice by acknowledging what we feel. Much energy is used being in urgency, and it is really a way to avoid feeling. When we avoid feeling by being busy, we create anxiety in our system. It is hard to be creative when we are anxious. So being less anxious is desirable on many levels. We can create a measurable increase in creativity when we breathe and calm our systems. Creativity allows us to be innovative and see the bigger picture, giving another perspective and it is possible for us all.

Can you recall the last time you were feeling very busy?
How did you manage this?
Would you like to explore another way?

Breathing is a simple and effective tool for dealing with busyness. We tend towards shallow breath when we are anxious, and it reminds us to slow down and acknowledge what we are feeling. Shallow breathing can become habitual. We may not even be aware we are breathing so shallowly. Holding the breath for short periods, rather than breathing in a relaxed, continuous cycle, is another way we can remain in an anxious state and avoid feeling. In my experience, I became aware I was shallow breathing to try and control my surroundings and not feel what was presenting. The illusion that we can control our surroundings by exerting a force against the natural ebb and flow of the universe is an interesting one. I found this just used considerable amounts of energy that wasn't available for other, more loving pursuits. When I became more conscious of how I habitually shallow breathed, I focused my attention on breathing differently. It took focused attention to do this as I had been shallow breathing and holding my breath for many years. Consistent effort over a period of time, learning to accept rather than control my environment changed my experience. I could choose to breathe more deeply in many more moments, allowing the feeling to present and move through as I stopped trying to block my feelings or judge them. The contraction in my system eased. When I learnt a new way I felt freed, and many of the physical aches and pains gradually disappeared. I was no longer locking up energy in my physical body in an effort to suppress my feelings. We have the choice of how we respond to all our experiences, and remembering that is key.

Consciously taking a deep breath and feeling life-force flooding through our being is a very simple tool that can be used moment after moment no matter what else is going on. This nurtures us at a deep level, connecting us with the love that resides at our core as an aspect of creation.

How does it feel to take a deep breath and keep breathing in an even and circular rhythm?

There was something else I used to spend time doing. I spent a lot of time thinking about what could go wrong and so was projecting into the future possible alternative realities that I didn't want to create. Our minds don't understand the difference between what we have actually experienced as opposed to what we are just thinking about, so I was creating realities I did not desire without any awareness of what I was doing. What we focus our attention on is what we create. Our thoughts are powerful, and even more so when spoken, as they then become energetic streamers or cords of energy that connect and are tangibly experienced by others.

Consider how we experience the words of others, both to wound and to uplift and inspire.

How often are we aware of the words we are using and the impact we are having on others and our environments?

So we not only create our own realities with what we think and say but we also impact others around us in loving or not so loving ways. Choosing the impact we will have requires Courage. We need to become aware of what we are thinking, saying and doing, honestly review our behavior and set our intention to do something different next time. Then we review that behavior and so on. Our lives are then about continuous review and improvement in the moment.

I used to get caught up in other people's urgencies as I didn't understand how to protect myself energetically. In this state, I was not very productive, but I thought I was doing pretty well. Much of my energy was directed towards what I didn't want rather than focused on what I wanted to achieve. I was clear what I didn't want, so could sense this in a more tangible way. For this reason, most of us are very good at being clear what we don't want and are moving away from and much less clear about what we would like to create. This is why many of us struggle to create goals with clear action steps towards achieving them. When we consider what we do want and move towards this step by step, we can be amazed by what we achieved. We are limited only by our own beliefs about what is possible. We are capable of so much more than our lower minds can grasp.

Moving towards what we value, being committed to continuous

self-development requires being really present in every moment. This is more than mindfulness, as we engage not just the mind in this but all of our Being. When we are clear on what we value, we can maintain our alignment.

Being aligned means connecting to our higher Self, choosing our focus and what we give our energy to. We may like to visualize this as a column of golden light that extends way above our head connecting with the bigger essence of who we are, while feeling the heart at the center as we connect into the earth way beneath our feet, anchoring into her core. Feel and see this column of continuous golden light surrounding us and within us in as many moments as we choose. This allows us to consider in more moments, whether we are moving closer to our values or farther away, towards the fear bandwidth. Can you feel the simplicity in this as life becomes clearly about choices and consequences? This allows us to maintain attention on what is important to us, and we can constantly monitor our progress.

Endurance assists us in moments of distraction. Monitoring and reviewing is very helpful in creating new awareness and making different choices. There is a wonderful simplicity in this. Can you feel the potential in experiencing life in this way?

Until we learn to trust the heart's knowing, we will be ruled by the lower mind, thinking in separation, cut off from the divine intelligence that the heart can access. In this limitation of the lower mind, we believe we are separate and everything is a potential threat. This produces fear and anxiety in our systems but there is another way.

Courage is the will to love, so we need to embrace uncertainty and another sacred quality: Adaptability. Courage is to feel the fear and do it anyway. There are really only two choices: love and fear. Love is simply the higher vibration of fear. We can all learn how to transform fear into love, with the application of simple tools used consistently. We need Courage to move forward in the face of fear. Without the sacred qualities of Courage and Endurance, we won't travel far on the path as love pioneers. Persistence in the face of adversity and resistance both from within and without can be reframed as just another opportunity to choose a more loving way.

Be still and listen to the heart; trust the quiet voice within to choose its own knowing.

Chapter 10

Transforming Nursing Practice

The best and most beautiful things in the world cannot be seen or even touched. They must be felt with the heart.
~ Helen Keller

Nurses are searching for new ways to transform their practice, knowing that the old ways no longer work.

The changes in nursing practice, a growing number of patients who want to be part of their recovery, a shrinking health budget and nurses who want to practice without feeling exhausted and disempowered are creating pressure for change. This can bring a sense of conflict and confusion as we tend to fear the unknown and try to hold on to what we know. This struggle goes on within each of us as we all hear the call of a distant voice, urging us to be more, to return home to our heart's knowing. The heart urges us to expand and question what we believe. To constantly challenge ourselves to contribute positively to our world requires us to quieten the other, the voice of the inner critic, that tells us we can't. This part of us seeks to maintain the status quo, to hold back, to contract, to limit.

However, we all have a choice about which voice we will listen to.

Which voice will we allow to direct our lives? Choosing to embrace a new way is possible for us all. It is not for the select few.

Our lower minds rationalize that the status quo is just fine, even if it is redundant, because we have allowed the lower mind to make the choices that seemingly keep us safe. But this is illusion, as living in fear and contraction attracts more of the same. It is only in surrendering to the heart that we find freedom—the freedom to not be constrained by fear and self-imposed limitation.

Surrendering to the new requires Adaptability and a desire to continually challenge self, remembering that there is a better way. We know that the only certainty is change, so letting go of the past is the only way to build the new. Nature lives this understanding through a constant cycle of birth, death and renewal, without getting in the way of itself, wishing it were summer when it is winter. The wisdom of the natural world has much to teach us about Surrender and Acceptance, flowing with what is and making the best of what presents. We are a part of the natural world and, as humans, we have the responsibility to play our part in evolving as nature does, in a continual state of renewal.

Feeling into our connection with some of the other kingdoms— the mineral kingdom: the rocks, soil, crystals, the plant kingdom, the animal kingdom—we can sense the Oneness as we remember we are not really separate. The pain of believing we are separate is an illusion. There is no separation as we tend to imagine, this exists only in our lower minds. Our minds are not the centers we have come to believe. It is our hearts that hold the key to transformation, personally and professionally. We are each responsible for our energetic being—each of us drops in the ocean, unique, but each creating the sea together; and this is where our strength lies: in playing our part, creating a tapestry of unique threads, producing something beautiful.

It takes Courage to step into the unknown, without a map, and trust the guidance we receive from the heart, acting when the opportunity presents. Having a mentor to champion us, to believe in us when we doubt ourselves, to acknowledge our growth can make all the difference to ongoing success.

A mentor who is on the path of heart mastery can't do it for us but they can walk beside us, encouraging, supporting and challenging as we find our way. We are all graced with opportunities every day, some major choices appearing like a fork in the road, and we consider what to do next.

We often understand that timing is important, as doors are not held open to accommodate procrastination, so this can add tension, creating urgency and vacillation. We must trust the heart's knowing rather than asking the mind, which will come up with all kinds of excuses why it isn't right for us or we don't have the skills or we are too busy. Being present and aware in more moments allows us to discern the most loving choice from our heart's knowing. Pondering in the heart rather than thinking about decisions produces very different results. It is a learnt skill we all know but have forgotten.

Feelings are the eyes of the heart and lead us to the truth. Feelings are experienced in all of our bodies and a healthy emotional state is dependent on allowing feelings to flow constantly. This helps us understand we don't need to be controlled by our emotional body. The emotional body becomes overwhelmed if we jam up feelings, creating states of dysfunction or shutting down our emotional body, effectively freezing it. We can change the state of our being by feeling what we feel instead of blocking it, denying it, storing it in our physical body—causing disease—or being overwhelmed by what we experience in our emotional body, impacting our ability to respond with emotional maturity.

We can learn to take responsibility for all of us by honoring what we feel, acknowledge feeling, releasing the judgment and choosing a higher vibration of expression. It is simple and if practiced with diligence, will create a new way of being for us all—impacting our teams, our patients, our organizations. We can then teach others by sharing the benefits we have experienced. Living life free from the struggle of pretending to be something we are not—expressing as full-bodied Beings—may feel new, but it is as old as time, as we come to know the Truth, uncovering the ancient knowledge that has been veiled.

This is an opportunity to experience life in a fuller sense, aligned with Truth and Grace, as we allow ourselves to be transformed into the full expression of our humanness, having a profound impact in our own lives, the lives of our patients and the organizations we work within.

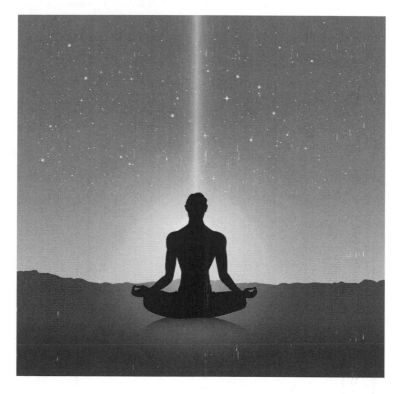

AYNI
BOOKS

"Ayni" is a Quechua word meaning "reciprocity" – sharing, giving and receiving – whatever you give out comes back to you. To be in Ayni is to be in balance, harmony and right relationship with oneself and nature, of which we are all an intrinsic part. Complementary and Alternative approaches to health and well-being essentially follow a holistic model, within which one is given support and encouragement to move towards a state of balance, true health and wholeness, ultimately leading to the awareness of one's unique place in the Universal jigsaw of life – Ayni, in fact.